Advance Praise

"Sylvester and Scherer are two master clinicians whose perspectives harmonize around practical and actionable ideas for clinicians and families. They explain complex topics in straightforward and no-nonsense terminology so that you don't have to wade through jargon or settle with feel-good cliché. Their lived experience comes through as two non-shaming voices that can be trusted to guide clinicians through the significant challenge of helping highly strained children and families connect today. The format of the book leads the reader deeper into walking the walk, as they learn to integrate both the neuroscience and the art of effective, compassionate treatment. This is a must-read for children and family therapists and should be on the reading list in graduate schools everywhere."

—**Sue Marriott**, LCSW, CGP psychotherapist and coproducer of Therapist Uncensored Podcast, a show consistently ranked in the Top 10 Social Science podcasts in the US and abroad

"Elizabeth Sylvester and Kat Scherer have created a readable gem for anyone helping families flourish. It teaches how to integrate neurobiology, attachment theory, emotional regulation, and relationship-based discipline into powerful, helpful interventions to support and guide families. Their conclusion says it well: *'Our hope is that this integrated perspective, and the concrete steps you can take to work within it, will be your takeaway . . .'* It's a book that will help you be a better therapist."

—**Kirke Olson**, PsyD, psychologist, school psychologist, and author of *The Invisible Classroom: Relationships, Neuroscience & Mindfulness in School*

"In *Relationship-Based Treatment of Children and Their Parents* Sylvester and Scherer skillfully summarize current wisdom regarding neurobiology, attachment, and regulation in relation to child development and parenting. Grounded in this context, they share details of the Nurtured Heart Approach, a straightforward relational framework for mindfully enhancing parent–child connections and supporting effective learning and boundary setting. Their warm and genuine style and inclusion of brief, personal examples to illustrate key points help to make the material relatable and accessible to students of family therapy. This book is a welcome addition for anyone seeking to set up family therapists, parents, and children for success!"

—**Cathy L. Cummings**, MA, PhD, program manager, Children's System of Care Training & Technical Assistance, Rutgers University Behavioral Health Care, Behavioral Research & Training Institute

"I created the Nurtured Heart Approach for parents who needed a better relational template to support challenging children to direct their intensity toward greatness. This book integrates the Nurtured Heart Approach with attachment theory and interpersonal neurobiology in an elegant, scholarly, and approachable way that therapists can immediately apply to working with children and families. I am so excited that therapists will have this compilation of Sylvester and Scherer's wisdom and experience to guide them in their work."

—**Howard Glasser**, creator, developer, and author of *The Nurtured Heart Approach*

RELATIONSHIP-BASED TREATMENT OF CHILDREN & THEIR PARENTS

The Norton Series on Interpersonal Neurobiology

Louis Cozolino, PhD, Series Editor

Allan N. Schore, PhD, Series Editor, 2007–2014

Daniel J. Siegel, MD, Founding Editor

The field of mental health is in a tremendously exciting period of growth and conceptual reorganization. Independent findings from a variety of scientific endeavors are converging in an interdisciplinary view of the mind and mental well-being. An interpersonal neurobiology of human development enables us to understand that the structure and function of the mind and brain are shaped by experiences, especially those involving emotional relationships.

The Norton Series on Interpersonal Neurobiology provides cutting-edge, multidisciplinary views that further our understanding of the complex neurobiology of the human mind. By drawing on a wide range of traditionally independent fields of research—such as neurobiology, genetics, memory, attachment, complex systems, anthropology, and evolutionary psychology—these texts offer mental health professionals a review and synthesis of scientific findings often inaccessible to clinicians. The books advance our understanding of human experience by finding the unity of knowledge, or consilience, that emerges with the translation of findings from numerous domains of study into a common language and conceptual framework. The series integrates the best of modern science with the healing art of psychotherapy.

RELATIONSHIP-BASED TREATMENT OF CHILDREN & THEIR PARENTS

AN INTEGRATIVE GUIDE TO NEUROBIOLOGY, ATTACHMENT, REGULATION, AND DISCIPLINE

ELIZABETH SYLVESTER • KAT SCHERER

FOREWORD BY DANIEL J. SIEGEL

Norton Professional Books

An Imprint of W. W. Norton & Company
Celebrating a Century of Independent Publishing

Copyright © 2023 by Elizabeth Sylvester and Kat Scherer
Foreword copyright © 2023 by Daniel J. Siegel

For information about permission to reproduce selections from this book, write to Permissions, W. W. Norton & Company, Inc., 500 Fifth Avenue, New York, NY 10110

For information about special discounts for bulk purchases, please contact W. W. Norton Special Sales at specialsales@wwnorton.com or 800-233-4830

Manufacturing by Versa Press
Production manager: Gwen Cullen

ISBN: 978-1-324-03056-0

W. W. Norton & Company, Inc., 500 Fifth Avenue, New York, NY 10110
www.wwnorton.com

W. W. Norton & Company Ltd., 15 Carlisle Street, London W1D 3BS

1 2 3 4 5 6 7 8 9 0

Contents

Foreword

BY DANIEL J. SIEGEL, MD

As a mental health practitioner working with children and parents, you may often find yourself challenged with how to effectively bring current views of relationships, development, and the process of change into your clinical approach. Elizabeth Sylvester and Kat Scherer are therapists who have immersed themselves in the world of interpersonal neurobiology, which combines various disciplines into a practical and science-based framework that can guide you toward effective evaluation and treatment for the families in your care. In *Relationship-Based Treatment of Children and Their Parents,* you'll find clear, science-informed explanations about the brain and self-regulation, emotional development and attachment, and the practical strategies of parental discipline and self-understanding that can all inform your work with families.

Offering an exciting way of diving deeply into these topics, our able guides demonstrate how to weave this knowledge and orient us to its practical implications, show examples of how this process works in ideal situations compared to challenging conditions, and then explore how to apply treatment interventions for effective implementation of these ideas. You'll learn about the science of attachment and its discoveries of how the relationship between child and caregiver shapes the function and structure of the child's developing brain. Attachment of child to parent, for example, shapes the child's regulatory capacities for emotion, memory, and behavior. At the same time, how parents understand how their own attachment experiences when they were children is the research-proven best predictor of how their own children will become attached to them. The good news about this empirical finding is that while we cannot change our own attachment history, we can change how we make sense of that history: understanding the ways the past impacted us, how we developed attachment strategies of survival, and then how we moved into our own adult life with these attachment states of mind.

By learning about the four basic strategies of attachment that developmental research has elucidated, as a clinician you will be offered a scientific framework for understanding and applying knowledge about attachment to clinical interventions. Knowing how secure attachment involves a "coherent narrative" and how the individual has made sense of the impact of the past on their present life can help you free them to be the parent they want to be. In contrast, having a history of emotionally disconnected parenting and the development of an avoidant attachment (and now a Dismissing state of mind with respect to attachment) in the adult may involve your using a different approach to clinical work; helping that parent get in touch with their own inner life and therefore the inner life of the child—to cultivate their "mindsight" abilities—in order to reflect on the mental world of self and others. For those with a history of intrusive and inconsistent parenting, the subsequent ambivalent attachment (and its Preoccupied state of mind in adulthood) may require a different way of supporting the adult in learning to regulate intense attachment needs that feel unfulfilled and fill them with sometimes overwhelming emotions. And those with a history of terrifying experiences with their caregivers may have developed disorganized attachment in childhood (and may now have an adult Unresolved state of mind). Their work would necessitate resolving the common history of trauma as abuse or loss with its frequent experience of dissociation.

You can sense from this brief overview of attachment science that how we adapt to our relationships early in life directly impacts the development of the mind's capacity to regulate our emotions, our thinking, and our behavior. In this way, the next section of the book is a natural shift to focusing on emotion, stress, and regulation, exploring how we can shift our "windows of tolerance" and help families learn to monitor and modify their own emotional communication and inner states. Louis Pasteur once said that "Chance favors only the prepared mind," and here our guides prepare our minds to help families by linking relational communication with inner regulation. Our minds are both embodied and relational, and as a mental health practitioner this realization is given practical application as you learn the science and art of how to nurture more effective means of communicating to promote an integrated brain at the heart of optimal regulatory capacity. Interpersonal integration leads to internal integration which is the basis for regulation—from emotion and thought to memory and morality.

As we then come to the third powerful part of this wonderful book, you'll see how parenting is an opportunity to teach, which is what the term "discipline" really means. Challenging moments in parenting can be reframed as opportunities for deep learning. Here you'll find a natural progression of your skills and knowledge from attachment science and brain aspects of regulation to parenting approaches that facilitate deep and lasting learning in children as they grow their autonomous skills for optimal regulation. With clinical examples of how to apply these ideas in working with families, this part continues to weave ideas and interventions in a creative and effective manner that will help you make this material your own framework, starting right as you finish each page, toward a science-grounded way of helping families function in a new way as they grow toward resilience and security.

As part of our professional series on interpersonal neurobiology, this book provides an important and practical guide to applying cutting-edge science to clinical work. Relationships are as much biology as the brain's neural circuits. When we learn the art of communication that enables energy and information flow to be shared between the attachment figure, the parent, and the developing child, we can see how the adage, "Where attention goes, neural firing flows, and neural connection grows" can support your clinical work to help cultivate integration in the relationship that is the basis of secure attachment, which is the basis of optimal regulatory abilities.

This wonderful guide will teach you the art and science of cultivating integration, inside and out—and it will be a gift that keeps on giving. Thank you for your devotion to children and their caregivers. Thank you for supporting families in becoming the nurturing safe haven and solid launching pad that enable children to grow well, become resilient, and be ready to face this challenging world we all live in.

Acknowledgments

This book would not have been written without the insights so freely offered by two groundbreaking creators and big-picture thinkers, Daniel Siegel and Howard Glasser. Their teachings and collegiality gave us a foundation on which to build, and the confidence to embark on this journey. We owe a debt of gratitude to our friends and colleagues, Richard Holt, Sue Marriott, and Al Scherer, who did the tedious work of reading early versions of the manuscript, and then kindly helped us clarify our message and find our voice. Our heartfelt thanks to our editor, Melissa Lowenstein, who was unwavering in her attunement and encouragement as we took our first steps toward publication. Her enthusiasm and patient, respectful suggestions were indispensable in making our work presentable. Warm acknowledgment to our parents and grandparents, and all of our lineage of parents, each generation building on the prior to lift up the next. This book is dedicated to our families, our partners, and children, who have been our ardent supporters over many years. Much love to Jeffrey, Jacob, Joshua, Ethan, Niels, and Eva; we are grateful for your constant and indispensable presence. And finally to our clients, who come for healing, but leave having taught and inspired us with their courage and wisdom. If you are reading this book, please know you have sparked these pages.

Book Organization and Structure

This book contains an introduction, Part I (Relationship-Based Treatment: Foundation in Science), and three major parts addressing attachment, emotion, and discipline (Part II, Attachment Foundations; Part III, Emotion, Stress, and Regulation; and Part IV, Transforming Behavior and Discipline).

Part I serves as a foundational introduction to and overview of the book. Parts II, III, and IV are each divided into four sections: first, an exploration of the theory and science of the topic; second, an illustration of what health and well-being might look like when things are going right—the ideal scenario; third, an exploration of family patterns when things are out of balance or going poorly—problem scenarios; and finally, a description of recommended treatment interventions. Each part of this book builds on the previous parts, to create a rich and integrative approach to child and family treatment.

Introduction

> Never doubt that a small group of thoughtful, committed citizens
> can change the world: indeed, it's the only thing that ever has.
> MARGARET MEAD, ATTRIBUTION IN DONALD KEYS,
EARTH TO OMEGA

It is an extraordinary group of individuals who focus their life's work on helping children and families. Working with families requires high levels of energy and patience, as well as an assured quality of hope. Therapists who become competent in transforming family patterns leave a legacy that betters the next generation.

Family therapists have many treatment approaches and techniques from which to choose. The mountain of scientific research, clinical data, and therapeutic strategies available can be mind-boggling and confusing. In this book, we review and integrate treatment options from highly respected sources to offer a consolidated approach to family treatment. Our approach gives a foundation for understanding presenting concerns and family patterns and targeting them with specific therapeutic tools. These tools include the therapist's interventions, but also include interventions designed for parents to apply as they move toward what we call relationship-based parenting.

Children and families burdened with attachment disruption, emotional distress, or psychological disorders need effective and immediate assistance.

They do not have the time to wait for long-term interventions or developmental changes to improve the parent–child relationship. Our experience suggests that the most effective approach in such situations includes interventions that impact the entire family at relational, emotional, and cognitive–behavioral levels, and that give parents agency to have rapid therapeutic impact on their children's lives and well-being. This is the approach presented in this book.

While some therapists may not be comfortable with one or more of these treatment orientations, we have found that a blended approach, applied with consistency and warmth, has the best chance of being effective.

THE FOUR CRITICAL AREAS OF STUDY FOR CHILD AND FAMILY THERAPISTS

Over decades of psychological study, clinical experience, and professional teaching, we have concluded that our therapeutic work is most robust when we apply an integrated approach. This book integrates four distinct areas of psychology: neurobiology, attachment theory, emotion, and relationship-based discipline (Figure I.1).

Neurobiology offers an understanding of our basic human foundation,

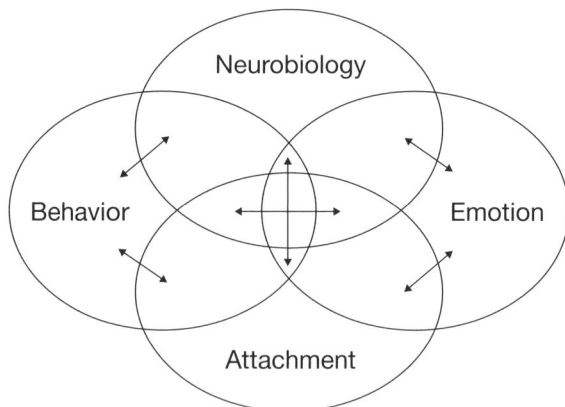

Figure I.1   Integrative Parenting

capacities, and needs. It describes how children develop biologically and provides research-based frameworks for understanding when specific abilities are available to them, including clarity about the ways in which neurological functions change when children feel safe versus when they are under stress. We focus on *interpersonal neurobiology*, a rich source of scientific knowledge, to describe how neurobiology shapes social and emotional experience, as well as how experience impacts neurological functioning (Siegel, 2020).

Attachment theory is rooted in over 70 years of theory and clinical research on our human social needs (Ainsworth et al., 1978; Bowlby, 1952, 1969; Cozolino, 2014; Karen, 1998; Main, 1990, 2006; Schore, 2001, 2015; Tronick, 2007; Winnicott, 1964/1992). It focuses on specific qualities of the critical first relationship between child and parent and identifies relational patterns and healing possibilities throughout life. Attention to attachment quality at home and in the treatment process dictates the capacity of any intervention to be well-received and durable. We utilize attachment theory to refine all interventions and techniques.

Emotional regulation impacts all areas of child development. Parents who offer an emotionally compassionate and stable presence lay a foundation for children to form flexible and adaptive emotional skills. This foundation helps children develop abilities that lead to confidence, social skills, and emotional regulation rooted in their neurobiological and cognitive systems (Fonagy et al., 2010; Panksepp & Biven, 2012; Porges, 2011; Schore, 2012, 2017; Siegel, 2020). An emotionally supportive home is also critical to the formation of secure attachments and effective relationship-based parenting.

Relationship-based discipline approaches are backed by applied research. They offer specific tools to facilitate relationship building, soothe painful emotions, and shape child behaviors into more functional patterns. The relationship-based approach we prefer is the Nurtured Heart Approach®, which is easy to grasp, consistent with neurobiology, and sound from an attachment perspective (Glasser & Easley, 2016; Glasser & Lowenstein, 2017; Hektner et al., 2013).

Each of these separate areas of theory and research can stand alone in the treatment of children and families. Combined, they offer a broad, deep, and powerful perspective that can directly enrich clinical practice.

Family therapists are in a unique position to bring this powerful integration to life in their work with parents and their children. The interweaving of neurobiology, attachment research, emotion, and relationship-based discipline produces a clear point of entry for therapists working with struggling families and provides interventions that are logical, doable, and highly effective.

RELATIONSHIP-BASED

TREATMENT

OF CHILDREN &

THEIR PARENTS

PART I

RELATIONSHIP-BASED TREATMENT: FOUNDATION IN SCIENCE

Integration is a basic law of life; when we resist it, disintegration is the natural result, both inside and outside of us. Thus we come to the concept of harmony through integration.

NORMAN COUSINS, *THE CELEBRATION OF LIFE*

1

Theory and Science of Parenting

Across psychological theories, the relationship between child and parent is acknowledged as a powerful and enduring influence in a child's emotional life. Here we review and discuss the robust research and accrued theoretical wisdom of our clinical community regarding the parent–child relationship. Children's abiding developmental need for a heartfelt, secure relationship with their parents was seen and described by our foundational thinkers, and is still considered and examined by current scientists.

Our clinical approach presented here is based on this science, old and new, including (1) neurobiology, (2) attachment theory, (3) emotional regulation, and (4) relationship-based discipline. In addition to an overview of these areas, we introduce several unique and crucial threads that are woven throughout this book, including the *7 essential attachment needs*, which every intervention in this book seeks to satisfy; identifying parental disruptions and family stress that create obstacles throughout the process; the value of beginning with parents when working therapeutically on behalf of children; and the importance of providing care that is immediately effective.

The heart and work of parenting is where each of these topics comes together in a practical way. Our approach is to help parents meet children's needs with a balance of warm heart and firm work. We view the heart as the compassionate, connected, attuned, playful aspect of parenting. We view the work as the clarity-providing, limit-setting, steady aspect of parenting. To consistently accomplish the elements of both heart and work, we must help parents dedicate themselves to developing their relational skills and abilities, along with self-awareness, self-regulation, and boundaries. Neither heart nor work function at their best in isolation; it is their balanced integration that is key for effective parenting.

NEUROBIOLOGY

Neurobiology is the foundation of our psychology and the base upon which children build cognitive skills, emotional intelligence, social abilities, and behavioral patterns. It is also the base from which parents regulate themselves to do their best parenting.

The therapist's understanding of the neurobiology behind therapeutic decisions can be the difference between intervention success or failure. Interventions can succeed when they are neurobiologically sound. We can't be successful if we are working in opposition to innate biological systems.

The field of interpersonal neurobiology was introduced by Dan Siegel, MD, a child psychiatrist and clinical professor at the UCLA School of Medicine. In his transformative psychology text *The Developing Mind*, he describes how life experiences and relationships shape the development of the brain and mind (Siegel, 2020). His description of the mind was created through collaboration with scientists from various disciplines—including biology, psychology, sociology, mathematics, and computer science—and defines the mind as formed within the integrated and dynamic process between the nervous system, physiology, and the social world in which one lives. The mind is not just neural activity; it is a complex, interdependent system involving internal physiology and the external environment.

These concepts clarify that the needs of children go well beyond cognitive stimulation. Children also require healthy social, emotional, and physical environments to thrive. With an enriched growth experience containing secure family relationships, rich emotional experiences, positive physical sensations, and cognitive stimulation, children are best able to develop their multifaceted minds (Panksepp & Biven, 2012; Porges, 2011; Siegel, 2017, 2020).

Interpersonal neurobiology offers an optimistic perspective that the human nervous system is *neuroplastic*: It has the capacity to learn and grow throughout the life span. This neurological plasticity persists through the life span, confirming that humans have the potential for lifelong growth and repair—regardless of whether or not one was raised in a positive, nurturing environment. Neuroplasticity also supports the role of psychotherapy to help individuals and families connect in growth-oriented ways, heal from past wounds, and promote secure attachments. It is never too late to learn and grow (Cozolino, 2014; Cramer et al., 2011; Davidson & McEwen, 2012; Levine, 2015; Schore, 2012; Siegel & Bryson, 2012; Vance et al., 2010).

Throughout this book, we synthesize and elaborate on this hopeful science and concept of repair and growth. Chapter 2 covers in detail relevant neurobiology to support the family therapist in facilitating brain-wise parenting.

ATTACHMENT THEORY

John Bowlby developed *attachment theory* in the mid-20th century and by 1969 was publishing his observations and ideas. His inquiry into the nature of the mother–infant bond and the repercussions of the quality of this bond was met with skepticism by other professionals. In particular, his suggestions that children's future mental health and overall development are related to their early attachment experiences and patterns were widely opposed (Bowlby, 1951). However, decades of longitudinal research and clinical data have confirmed his conclusions that the quality of early attachment strongly shapes children's path of development into adulthood (Ainsworth et al., 1978; Bowlby, 1952, 1969; Brazelton & Greenspan, 2001; Brown & Elliott, 2016; Cozolino, 2014; Karen, 1998; Lester & Sparrow, 2010; Main, 1990, 2006; Schore, 2017; Tronick, 2007, 2017; Winnicott, 1964/1992). Attachment research over the past 65 years has expanded beyond the mother–infant relationship to include other important emotional bonds across the life span.

The decades of research on parent–child attachment have resulted in four validated categories of attachment: secure, ambivalent insecure, avoidant insecure, and disorganized. Individuals within a given attachment category have been found to have similar relational patterns in their adult lives. A secure early bonding relationship offers children the experience of primary trust and safety that lays the foundation for self-esteem, social confidence, and other benefits later in life. Security is likely to develop when the parent–child relationship is safe, reliable, and caring. Some scientists say attachment has the most substantial impact on the trajectory of children's development (Bowlby, 1969; Brazelton & Sparrow, 2006; Karen, 1998; Lester & Sparrow, 2010; Medina, 2014; Tronick, 2007; Winnicott, 1964/1992). In Part II of this book, we explore the science and applicable theory behind a healthy attachment connection and illustrate clinical processes that can enrich children's development.

EMOTIONAL REGULATION

In Part III, we focus on emotion, stress, and self-regulation. In children's early years, emotional awareness and adaptivity are evolving within the parent–child relationship at neurobiological and cognitive levels (Gross, 2014). Supportive emotional family experiences lay the foundation for future resiliency, social ease, and self-worth. Parents with emotional sensitivity and sympathy create an environment that recognizes all emotions, both positive and negative. Purposely acknowledging and attending to positive feelings creates the potential for children to experience hope and joy. Parental understanding and support in challenging situations offer children strength to cope with pain and suffering. Stress and struggles are part of life; how parents respond matters.

Secure parent–child relationships depend on emotional sensitivity, compassion, and attunement. Parental support helps children to develop the skills they need to cope with and work through difficult feelings such as sadness, anxiety, loss, or trauma. In an emotionally present home, children feel heard, understood, and accepted; they are not alone. Children are emotionally vulnerable and reactive by nature. Their immature feelings can sometimes enhance, and sometimes stress, a family system. Emotionally empathic and stable adults are critical supports for maturing children. In addition, these emotional connections are the foundation of secure attachments and are needed for the success of relationship-based parenting.

RELATIONSHIP-BASED DISCIPLINE

Children are sponges, continually learning at conscious and unconscious levels. This means that what parents do in relationship with their children really matters. They are the most powerful influence in most areas of children's growth, and the best equipped to promote health of all types in their children. Parents are formative as attachment figures, educators, and role models, whether they intend to be or not. Parents' mindfulness, sensitivity, and control over their own behavior are imperative for positive guidance and teaching to occur. And parents' effectiveness as sources of comfort and boundaries is inevitably determined by the quality of the relationship they are able to construct with their children.

All parenting approaches require parents to be aware and intentional with their children, and to cultivate self-awareness and emotion management. Parents' own self-control provides a critical foundation for a safe and reliable environment. However, since parents are human, they will make mistakes. They will be thoughtless at times. So parents' self-awareness and capacity to attend to relational repair are also components of a positive, dynamic parent–child relationship.

It is important to note that when we refer to discipline in this book, we do not equate it with negativity or punishment. *Discipline means teaching.* Its goal is to help children learn productively from their experiences and mistakes. For children to learn, they must feel emotionally safe and be cognitively open, and the lesson needs to fit their developmental level. This book discusses parenting with emotions and development in mind.

In Part IV, we discuss which parenting approaches are effective, which are not, and why. We share several concrete tools available to quickly shift negative family patterns toward positivity and growth.

THE NURTURED HEART APPROACH

Many popular parenting approaches are described in the literature. We favor the Nurtured Heart Approach (NHA) because it is relationship-focused, therapeutic, and compatible with neurobiological science and attachment theory (Hektner et al., 2013).

This approach, developed by Howard Glasser, is a relational approach designed to guide parents in their efforts to move children away from negative, self-defeating patterns and into positive, productive interactions with themselves and others. It effectively fosters emotional and behavioral regulation in a way that is neurobiologically consistent and attachment-sound.

The Nurtured Heart Approach is effective as a relationship-based intervention that potently decreases problematic behaviors in children (Nuño et al., 2020). Due to its focus on attunement, reflection, acceptance, and emotional safety, it has powerful cognitive and relational components. This approach has a positive impact on children's self-image and self-esteem and shifts family relationship patterns in a positive direction. It has been successfully used in homes, schools, and treatment settings to increase attachment security and decrease negative interactions.

SUPPORTING PARENTS TO MEET CHILDREN'S ESSENTIAL ATTACHMENT NEEDS

Our integrated approach evolved to provide a structure for family therapy work focusing on dynamic issues in complicated family relationships. In an ideal situation, parents have the physical and emotional resources to meet their children's developing needs; they offer a safe, caring, attentive, and boundaried home in which their children can flourish. It is not necessary for the home to be perfect; no home is. Parents can be what D. W. Winnicott (1953) called "the good enough parent" as long as they can, with relative consistency, provide certain qualities that have been found to facilitate children's health and family satisfaction.

The literature on child development offers many different perspectives on the basic needs of children to grow strong, healthy, and happy. We have integrated scientific research, developmental theory, and practical clinical experience to create a list of *7 essential attachment needs* of children for optimal development (Bowlby, 1969; Brazelton & Greenspan, 2001; Brazelton & Sparrow, 2006; Brown & Elliott, 2016; Cozolino, 2014; Karen, 1998; Lester & Sparrow, 2010; Schore, 2012, 2015; Siegel, 2020; Tronick, 2007; Winnicott, 1953; Winnicott, 1964/1992). When these foundational qualities are present, parents have created a favorable environment: fertile ground in which children can thrive. This list is both brain-wise and attachment sound.

THE 7 ESSENTIAL ATTACHMENT NEEDS

1. Safety and Security
2. Soothing
3. Attunement
4. Reliability and Consistency
5. Support and Encouragement
6. Stimulation, Novelty, and Fun
7. Boundaries and Structure

This list is elaborated throughout this book and serves as an aspirational guide for considering the strengths and weaknesses of a family system. The 7 essential attachment needs are a basis for appreciating parents' existing abilities and setting treatment goals for growing in underdeveloped areas (described in more detail in Chapter 4).

INTEGRATION OF THE DEVELOPING SELF

When children's fundamental needs are met, they have a safe place to experiment and process their world—to explore both their inner and outer lives. This freedom to be curious about themselves and the world facilitates learning and, over time, a comfortable awareness of all the facets of themselves, including their emotional, cognitive, and physical experiences. Such skills as problem solving and self-soothing grow from such integrated and accepting self-awareness. For example, children can learn to recognize signs from their thinking process or from their bodies that emotions are present and need their attention. They can learn to respond to their painful feelings by using positive thoughts to soothe themselves. They can self-soothe by seeking comfort from safe others and can regulate their stress through movement or productive behavior. Such integration of mind, body, and emotion is evidence of mental health.

According to Dr. Dan Siegel, families that provide well for their children's fundamental needs will create an optimal environment for integration of brain, body, and emotional processes. A result of such integration is the formation of positive qualities of flexibility, adaptability, coherence, energy, and stability (FACES; Siegel, 2020). A system integrated across neurological, physiological, cognitive, and emotional experiences is steadying, flexible, and associated with resilience (Brazelton & Greenspan, 2001; Brazelton & Sparrow, 2006; Lester & Sparrow, 2010; Medina, 2014; Siegel, 2015a, 2017; Schore, 2012; Ogden & Fisher, 2015; Ogden et al., 2006; van der Kolk, 2015).

PARENTING DISRUPTIONS AND COMPLICATIONS

Unfortunately, for many families, meeting the 7 essential attachment needs seems impossible. In our clinical work, we observe that families who struggle with meeting these needs experience repercussions in the quality of the parent–child relationship. The resulting disruptions often lead to chronic strain and discomfort in parenting that can create and perpetuate a negative cycle of emotional and relational disruption for children and families, as well as problems in children's development, if not corrected (Baylin & Hughes, 2016; Cozolino, 2014; Cramer et al., 2011; Davidson & McEwen, 2012; Karen, 1998; Parkes et al., 2006; Schore, 2001, 2015; Wallin, 2007; Winnicott, 1964/1992).

Family relationship complications can arise from a variety of factors such as a child's innate biological vulnerabilities, a child's early trauma or loss, a parent's history of adversity, or (more often) a mix of all the above. For example, children who are by nature (or temperament) unusually intense—who, emotionally or behaviorally, require very high levels of attunement, security, and structure—put greater demands on parents as they work to create a strong and stable relationship. Other children have experienced preexisting attachment disruptions from early histories of trauma or neglect, which can disrupt emotional bonding. Parents' own painful backgrounds of trauma or grief can make it more difficult for them to form secure emotional connections with their children.

Any of these challenges are compounded when families live under heavy environmental stresses including poverty, high-pressure jobs, dangerous neighborhoods, racism, or health issues. These added burdens can impact parents' ability to interact with children in an attachment-sound way. As a result, children may feel needy, frustrated, or tense, which can, in turn, create a pattern of withdrawal, demanding, or other behavioral acting out. In their turn, parents often respond with frustration, overwhelm, anger, or sadness. A negative and self-perpetuating cycle can then establish itself.

Problematic family situations can also create strong motivations and opportunities for positive change. Under these challenging conditions, the goal in family treatment is to break into the negative cycle and increase parents' ability to create and sustain a safe and stable relationship, even in the face of adversity. The development of a positive, stable parent–child connection can serve as a buffer against the negative forces in or around the family (Tronick, 2017).

BEGIN WITH THE PARENTS

When working on behalf of children and families, a therapist may choose to intervene using individual psychotherapy, parenting consultation, or family therapy. The perspectives offered in this book apply in any of these modalities.

The model we most often recommend begins with parenting work: meeting with the parents without children present. This approach allows parents to focus on making immediate family changes while reducing the likelihood of children feeling pathologized by being placed in treatment. In many cases, the necessary family system-wide shifts can be achieved by the parents alone making adjustments to their style of interaction with family members (Deblinger & Heflin, 1996).

Once parenting skills and habits have been addressed, the major work may be done. In cases where continued intervention is needed, family therapy or individual psychotherapy for the parent or child may be warranted.

THERAPIST–CLIENT DYNAMICS

It is essential to note that there are parallel dynamics in the therapist–client relationship. The quality of the therapeutic relationship is critical for treatment success. Parents look to the therapist for attributes of safety, reliability, and relief from suffering as they trust the therapist with intimate struggles in their family life. Therapists can build trust by making sincere efforts to understand the parents (attention and caring), by being reliable and consistent (predictable), and creating realistic treatment plans for positive change (hope). In every session, therapists have the opportunity to model security through their self-regulation, therapeutic efforts, and respectful boundaries, and through the building of a safe therapeutic environment. These qualities, along with the therapist's knowledge and confidence, increase the family's determination to engage in treatment (Laska et al., 2014; Wampold, 2017).

FAMILIES WITH URGENT NEEDS

When family dynamics interfere with the development of a strong parent–child bond, there is a great and immediate need for effective care. These families do not have the luxury of waiting for years of treatment or parent education to change their personal patterns or family milieu. A parent–child relationship that is not gratifying or feels excessively stressful can lead to chronic family tension. Under these conditions, parents need clear and doable guidelines to feel more confident and capable and to make the home environment immediately more secure and nurturing. An integrated understanding of neurobiology, attachment, emotion, and relationship-based discipline helps professionals efficiently guide parents to healthier patterns that increase children's sense of security, connection, and boundaries, and can rapidly decrease tension and negativity at home.

The science is conclusive: A positive and secure childhood enhances children's lives regardless of their circumstances. When parents are attentive, reliable, and caring, they lay the foundation for optimal physical, intellectual, and emotional development. Of course, environment, genetics, and temperament play a role, but primary attachments have a powerful influence on the path of growth. The primary relationship with parents shapes a child's growing brain, body, and heart. The good news is that families do not need to be perfect. Any movement in the right direction is helpful, and it is never too late to make positive changes in the family.

2

Neurobiology of Parenting: In Brief

Our goal in this chapter is to provide a concise and thorough review of the developmental neurology of children and the neurological patterns behind supportive and unsupportive behaviors of parents. We will introduce the following three elements, which are foundational information to support the parenting approach detailed in this book: (1) neurological development, (2) autonomic nervous system (ANS) and polyvagal theory, and (3) integration of neurological and biological systems.

A child's brain is amazing and always evolving. As children grow, their neurological development goes through some predictable phases that offer critical information about children's capacities and readiness for certain kinds of learning. Knowledge of age-related maturational trends in behavior will help therapists and parents develop realistic expectations for young children. Parents with accurate expectations will put energy where children need it the most and develop patience with their children's immature nervous systems.

NEUROLOGICAL FOUNDATIONS OF DEVELOPMENT

Humans are born with billions of neurons and a trillion weblike neural connections. In the first five years of life, there is an explosion of growth as our early experiences are literally encoded into our nervous systems. Learning starts before we are born and explodes in the first few years of life, adding to the structure and complexity of the child's brain.

A baby's brain creates 700 new neural connections every second. In the first year of life, the brain weaves 10 billion new interneuronal links per day. School-aged children can develop up to three times more neurons and interconnections than they will end up with as adults (Flaherty & Rost, 2011). Imagine brilliance or chaos; this is the brain of a child.

In the first five years, the primary foundation for most future learning is established. Over childhood and adolescence, the development of myelin sheaths around some neurons increases the brain's processing speed. In later childhood and adolescence, the neurological system develops the intricacy, sophistication, and efficiency required for higher-order adult learning and memory (see Table 2.1, as well as Part IV, Transforming Behavior and Discipline).

In adolescence, significant structural changes take place as neural connections are trimmed back, reorganized, and myelinated for efficiency (coordination and speed). During this period, some neurons die out and some links are broken. This process, called *neural pruning*, creates an opportunity to fine-tune and strengthen the growing brain (Andersen, 2003; Balocchini et al., 2013; Siegel, 2015; Spear, 2013; Strauch, 2004).

As you can imagine, this restructuring of the brain can temporarily weaken immature adolescent cognitive and emotional systems. The executive prefrontal cortex does not mature until the late 20s. If structural, genetic, or psychological problems exist, they may be revealed during this time of rapid change.

Ideally, neural pruning and restructuring will eventually improve cognitive skills and mental efficiency, and will create a simpler, stronger, and faster structure for adulthood. Across our lifespan, the integration of these neural networks builds further mental complexity and efficiency.

Table 2.1 INFANT TO ADULT GLOBAL NEUROLOGICAL DEVELOPMENT	
0–1 years	The right hemisphere of the brain—the predominant hemisphere in the process of building a primary attachment base—develops more quickly than the left.
0–4 years	Children develop a foundation for hearing, vision, language, and physical development from the brain's back and sides.
5–7 years	As the cerebral cortex and cerebellum grow, children make developmental leaps in terms of learning, social skills, and coordination.
8–12 years	In the preadolescent years, there is growth in memory and higher-order thinking as the frontal lobe makes a surge in development. The brain begins restructuring for complexity and efficiency.
13–19 years	In adolescence, the brain undergoes major neurological changes, pruning and rewiring neurons to create the foundation for a more efficient and integrated adult brain. Greater emotional lability is a typical consequence of rapid change in neuronal structures.
20–30 years	By the late 20s, neuronal maturation is complete. The prefrontal cortex—the seat of high-level thought, attention span, planning ability, self-reflection, self-control, and moral reasoning, necessary for rational thought and behavior—is among the last areas to mature.

"Neurons That Fire Together Wire Together" (*Hebb's rule*)

Research indicates that our brains have a natural ability to change and grow throughout the lifespan (Ang & Gomez-Pinilla, 2007; Cozolino, 2014; Cramer et al., 2011; Davidson & McEwen, 2012; Fisher et al., 2004; Petzinger et al., 2015; Schore, 2012; Siegel, 2020; Siegel & Bryson, 2012; Stegemoller, 2014; Vance et al., 2010). When an experience is repeated over time, a pattern of neuronal and chemical firing is formed in the nervous system. It literally creates pathways in the brain that, with repeated use, become well established—the route more likely to be taken. Hence, Hebb's rule: Neurons that fire together wire together.

This potential for lifelong neurological change is called neuroplasticity. We can rewire our brains for the better at any age, and parental guidance has a powerful influence on which neurons fire and what becomes wired into children's brains.

THE AUTONOMIC NERVOUS SYSTEM
AND REGULATION

The ANS is part of the peripheral nervous system, which regulates the activity of physiological processes that run outside of conscious awareness. It manages such actions as breathing, heart rate, blood flow, and digestion. It also controls human social engagement and the stress response and serves as the human safety system.

The ANS functions through two major sections: the *parasympathetic nervous system* (PNS), also known as the rest-and-digest system; and the *sympathetic nervous system* (SNS), the fight-or-flight system. When there is an extreme risk to safety, the *dorsal vagal portion of the PNS* can shift into an emergency state and immobilize the body, creating a faint or collapse response to ensure survival.

Mammalian physiology has evolved the ability to enjoy calm and social states when the environment is safe. This state is governed by the myelinated portion of the vagus nerve (ventral), which is the PNS's dampening system for the reactive and danger-sensitive SNS. It literally puts the brakes on our defensive system and allows us to be calm and open. Its job is to settle the human nervous system's historical (phylogenetic) tendency to be tense and alert for any hint of threat to personal safety. When allowed to run its course, the SNS is in a state of fight or flight, fear, or agitation, and is highly reactive and protective. In a PNS (ventral vagal) state, however, the body can relax, digest food, heal injuries, grow, and engage with others. This social and relaxed mode is the state in which humans are the most friendly, healthy, and happy. Ideally, this should be the primary state of the body.

When the environment is perceived as unsafe, the SNS works through a series of chemical changes in the body to release the stress hormones adrenaline and cortisol, which kick the body into action (fight or flight). These stress hormones increase heart rate, blood pressure, blood flow, muscle tension, and breath frequency and move blood flow away from nonessential functions such as digestion, reproduction, and growth. In this state, the human mind is not capable of attuned social connections. Hearing and vision changes related to the brain and body's focus on quickly securing safety make it difficult to communicate with someone in this state. Also, there is a temporary immobilization defense, called freeze, hypothesized to utilize the myelinated ventral vagal PNS brake, with sympathetic tone, to immobilize muscles during assessment of a threat just prior to a fight, flight, or faint response (Roelofs, 2017).

At another extreme, if the environment is perceived as threatening to one's life, the unmyelinated portion of the PNS (dorsal vagal) can shift the body into a state of immobilization collapse in a last-ditch effort to survive: the faint or feigning death response. This is an automatic reaction, not a conscious decision. This state can be dangerous due to a potentially dramatic drop in heart rate. Neither of these defensive states (SNS or dorsal vagal PNS response) allow for normal social engagement. It follows that when parents or children are in a defensive state, they are unable to access the social and emotional engagement skills needed for healthy relating.

After the threat subsides, the body should naturally shift back to the calm and socially engaged state of PNS (ventral vagal) control over the nervous system. In this state, relationships can repair and reconnect. Where stress is severe or chronic, however, SNS or dorsal vagal PNS systems remain active, potentially leading to physical and emotional problems such as cardiovascular disease, respiratory illnesses, immune deficiency, emotional dysregulation, depression, insomnia, and anxiety.

POLYVAGAL THEORY: EMOTIONAL REGULATION AND SOCIAL ENGAGEMENT

Polyvagal theory provides insight into why our social engagement varies from defensive or aggressive to friendly and sociable depending on the nervous system's perception of safety or danger in the moment (Porges, 2011). It posits that the vagus nerve, which runs from the brain to the gut, evolved in mammals to regulate social behavior and ensure safety. It is central to expression of emotions via body language, facial expression, and tone of voice, and to our ability to read those expressions in others. The vagus nerve influences one's sense of safety, mood, and body language, as well as heart rate, respiration, energy levels, and digestion. In psychotherapeutic work with families, information from polyvagal theory can promote understanding of the neurological underpinnings of their social and emotional interactions with one another (Porges, 2011, 2017; Porges & Furman, 2012).

When an individual is in a relaxed state and the newer PNS is active, the ventral vagal nerve is engaged, which puts a brake on one's innate defensive reactivity. This allows that person to cooperate and to be friendly and playful. In this state, family members are easily capable of empathy and care. However, when a person is triggered by a challenge or threat, they move into a hyperaroused SNS state. In this state, the ventral vagal brake is disengaged, and the person feels some level of anxiety or anger: anywhere from low levels of worry or irritation to high levels of panic or rage. This is the fight-or-flight response described above: the person either has an angry urge to attack or a fearful urge to run. In this state, the individual's ability for positive engagement with others is impaired. Cooperation and empathy are weak or absent as the person functions from a more self-centered, self-protective position.

If the threat persists, and the person's attempts to create safety through fight or flight fail, they can become overwhelmed by the stress of the ongoing threat. In these moments, the body mounts a last-ditch defense in which both the SNS and dorsal vagal PNS are activated, and the PNS dominates (Roelofs, 2017). In this emergency state, the dorsal vagal PNS inhibits the SNS fight-or-flight response; the person feels helpless, numb, dissociated, and shut down. This is the faint or collapse state, characterized by flat affect, diminished eye contact, and significantly decreased social behavior. As discussed above, an important detail of polyvagal theory is that one's vagal responses are not under voluntary control. A person does not choose to become defensive, self-protective, angry, frightened, or shut down. The body decides for us, and it decides instantly.

At any given moment, every individual has their own balance of SNS and dorsal/ventral vagal PNS activity, and this is reflected in their affect and relational actions. When a person feels safe and at ease (ventral vagal PNS dominant), their comfort is reflected in their relaxed body posture and facial expression, warm tone of voice, and eye contact. When a person feels threatened, angry, or frightened (SNS or dorsal vagal PNS), their stress shows up as physical rigidity or agitation, constricted vocal tone, limited eye contact, tense facial expression, or dissociation/collapse. These physical expressions reflect whether the person feels safe or unsafe, as well as sending a message to other people about the safety or unsafety of the environment in which they find themselves. The state of one person's nervous system directly affects the state of another person's nervous system. Our social interactions are contingent on these conscious and unconscious social signals.

One important goal of psychotherapy or parenting work is to open a window for personal awareness around the topic of self-regulation, which can then create positive relational change. Reading the cues in our own bodies that tell us how the other is feeling is the foundation of attunement, and parents can learn to do this with their children. The therapist's regulation of their own nervous system and awareness of others' emotional states is a critical aspect of treatment, in terms of both providing a calm, safe environment for therapy and modeling the self-regulation required to provide such an environment. Clients who feel truly relaxed and safe with the therapist are far more likely to engage with therapy in a productive manner. Parents can draw upon this same kind of emotional awareness to help them better connect with their children.

The astonishing and complex ANS has the fundamental goals of survival and connection. It is a system designed to keep ourselves and our children alive and safe. To this end, it has the built-in ability to detect safe and unsafe situations, to encourage connection with and reliance on safe others, and to motivate care for oneself and one's children. In families where SNS or dorsal vagal PNS responses are overfrequent, healthy functioning and relating become difficult. Individuals need to find a balance between the SNS/dorsal vagal and ventral vagal PNS states to create functional families.

Humans need both sides of the nervous system to work together flexibly and adaptively to create social relationships that are cooperative, productive, and safe. All of our best and most effective psychotherapy treatments should align with this aspect of basic human physiology and its fundamental human purposes: the cultivation of safety and connection.

INTEGRATION OF NEUROLOGICAL STRUCTURE AND FUNCTION

This section shifts away from the larger neurological system to focus on the specific functioning of the brain. Human brains are a combination of structures that, ideally, function as an integrated and interactive whole. The left and right hemispheres, the upper, middle, and lower brain structures, and other specialized regions of the brain with unique functions all work together, with support from integrative parts whose main purpose is to foster communication and integration between brain regions. This mental integration makes it possible for people to complete complex tasks, organize information, regulate physical and emotional responses, and respond productively and appropriately to new situations (Cozolino, 2014; Dubuc, 2013; Menon & Uddin, 2010; Porges, 2011; Schore, 2015; Siegel, 2017, 2020; Snyder et al., 2011; Taylor et al., 2008; Tiemeier et al., 2010). In the following sections, we focus on the roles of individual brain regions, with full recognition that these regions do not work independently of one another.

The Horizontal Brain: The Right and Left Hemispheres

The brain's cortex is composed of the right and left hemispheres, connected by a network of neural fibers in the center of the brain called the *corpus callosum* (Figure 2.1). The corpus callosum inhibits either the left or right hemisphere, allowing one or the other to dominate depending on what function is primarily needed at the time.

The right side of the brain is often described as the holistic and creative brain and the left side as linear, logical, and language oriented. The right brain tends to be more visual-spatial and emotional; it recognizes others' faces, interprets nonverbal communication, and assigns meaning. The left brain is more language and math based, driven to explain things. During the first year of life, the baby's right hemisphere—which is focused on attachment, a form of social connection—is dominant and growing rapidly.

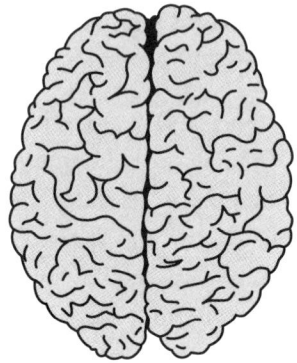

Figure 2.1   The Horizontal Brain: Hemispheres

Some adults tend to appear more right-brained or left-brained in their thinking style, with either logic or creativity predominant; but to optimally use memory, logic, and creativity, we need both sides of the brain. In Iain McGilchrist's *The Master and His Emissary*, he describes the right brain as the master and the left brain as its faithful servant. He observes that our society has tended to honor the "servant"—the linear and logical—at the expense of the "sacred gift" of our right brain, the holder of creativity and intuition. Also, our educational systems have tended to favor the linear and logical (McGilchrist, 2012). In the end, however, the left and right hemispheres need each other, just as Sherlock and Watson need each other to be successful and complete.

The Vertical Brain: Brain Stem, Limbic System, and Cerebral Cortex

The brain is also organized vertically, with lower, middle, and upper regions. The lower brain is composed of the brain stem; the middle brain is the limbic system; and the upper brain is the cerebral cortex, including our highest-order functions in the prefrontal cortex (Figure 2.2). For our purposes in this book, we will primarily focus on the limbic system and the highly evolved prefrontal cortex.

The limbic system is in the middle of the brain, with the amygdala and the hippocampus, which compose our personal security and defensive reaction system. When the limbic system senses potential danger, it facilitates the release of stress hormones to prepare us to seek safety. The prefrontal cortex, on the other hand, is in the upper frontal portion of the brain and houses our highest-order thinking skills, which are needed for cognitive, social, and emotional development. This region includes our executive functioning such as self-awareness, social sensitivity, emotional regulation, attention span, planning abilities, and self-control (Table 2.2).

Many regions of young children's brains are not yet fully developed, which limits their abilities. The prefrontal cortex is last to complete development, finishing in the late 20s. This immaturity limits the capacity for impulse control, attention, and emotional regulation for children, teenagers, and young adults.

However, this is a two-way system. The reactive limbic system can also send anxious or defensive signals to the cortex, which can trigger negative thought cycles of fear or anger, which in turn can activate the stress response. Also, when individuals are stressed, hungry, or tired, they are more likely to act from the limbic, reactive, or defensive systems. This state of mind is likely to arise during family conflict.

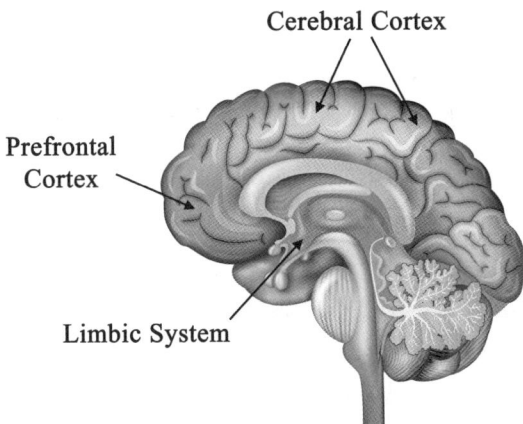

Figure 2.2 The Vertical Brain SOURCE: © Gunita Reine/Depositphotos.com

Table 2.2		
Limbic System **Middle Brain**	**Cerebral Cortex** **Upper Brain**	**Prefrontal Cortex** **Upper Front Brain**
Memory	Memory (explicit)	Executive functions:
Emotion	Emotion	Attention
Motivation	Sensory input	Reflection
Drive	Movement	Decision making
Equilibrium	Language	Planning
Autonomic functions	Abstract thought	Impulse control
	Creativity	Emotion regulation
		Prosocial behavior
		Moral reasoning

Fortunately, when thoughts and feelings are brought back into a state of calm, we can better resolve conflict and emotionally reconnect. We do our best thinking and emotion regulation in states of calm. When relaxed and secure, parents and children are better able to access the higher-order brain (prefrontal cortex) to consciously regulate and integrate thoughts, feelings, compassion, and past experiences.

INTEGRATION FOR WELL-BEING

The human brain and nervous system are complex, ever-shifting, and incredible. This system develops naturally on a biologically determined and predictable path, while also being heavily influenced by the surrounding environment. Family culture saturates the developing mind, informing it about what states, feelings, and behaviors are acceptable and useful.

As discussed earlier, the secure child–parent relationship provides a nurturing environment in which a child can safely experience and integrate their neurological, physiological, emotional, and cognitive systems. The goal throughout childhood is to develop, in the context of a supportive family, qualities of adaptability, integrity, strength, and cohesion. According to

Dan Siegel (2020), this process is the foundation of a strong sense of self, social development, and overall feelings of well-being.

This dynamic developmental process, enveloped with security and nurturance, can help children develop optimal growth and integration across their physical and emotional systems (Brazelton & Greenspan, 2001; Brazelton & Sparrow, 2006; Gross, 2014; Lester & Sparrow, 2010; Medina, 2014; Schore, 2012; Siegel, 2015; Ogden et al., 2006; van der Kolk, 2015). This strong foundation creates an environment where children can develop strength and adaptability.

Meeting children's essential attachment needs helps set the stage for proper integration of all the parts of the brain. It creates a foundation for well-rounded development, smooth linking of brain, body, and emotion, and eventual neurological integration and maturity. In Part II, we dive deeply into the foundations and implications of early childhood attachment.

PART II

ATTACHMENT FOUNDATIONS

The truth is that from the day we are born until the day we die we need to feel held and contained somewhere. We can let go and become independent only when we feel sufficiently connected to other people.

R. TAFFEL, *PARENTING BY HEART*

3

Orientation to Theory and Science: Children's Essential Attachment Needs

Throughout modern history, experts on children's health have been committed to a parade of different perspectives on child-rearing. Strategies based on these perspectives have been pressed on parents to equip them to meet children's fundamental needs. As civilization has rapidly evolved over the past hundred years, those needs have evolved as well, as have recommended strategies for parenting in ways that maximize the chances that children will get what they need to survive and thrive.

A hundred years ago, when infectious illness was the paramount threat to babies and young children, well-meaning professionals placed heavy emphasis on cleanliness, sterile environments, and keeping children safe through protection from infection. This led to a general practice of keeping physical distance from children and more extreme methods of isolation of sick children from their parents. Orphaned children were warehoused in clean but relationally barren environments.

Into this milieu stepped John Bowlby in the 1940s, with his then-revolutionary perspective that warmth, physical affection, and emotional attunement are critical for healthy child development. He faced an ugly and uphill battle against established theory and conventional wisdom. In retrospect, his insights seem obvious; at the time, they were radical. Today, knowing that Bowlby was right, it is painful to look back on films such as *A Two-Year-Old Goes to Hospital* (Robertson & Robertson, 1952) or *Emotional Deprivation in Infancy* (Spitz, 1952)—coldly clinical, real-life illustrations of the devastating impact of parent–child separation and lack of emotional connection and safety.

From our current position, it is easy to feel proud of our progress and confident in our perspectives. Yet we should not be resting on our laurels; much work remains to be done. It is incumbent upon us to continue to expand our understanding of our intellectual inheritance around the topic of child-rearing. We must stay humble to the fact that we are lodged in our history and that we are not above perpetuating its errors.

THE LIFELONG IMPACT OF ATTACHMENT

As Bowlby emphasized, we are social beings by nature, and there is enormous power in our relational drive. When we receive the connection we crave, we thrive. When it is absent, we suffer, and damage occurs. For our youngest patients, healthy early attachment relationships lay the foundation of social and emotional development. Warm and reliable parents build trust and the expectation of positivity in relationships. This is the heart of parenting.

This security plays out across life with documented results of stronger resiliency, relational capacity, and confidence (Brazelton & Greenspan, 2001; Cozolino, 2014; Karen, 1998; Lester & Sparrow, 2010; Schore, 2017; Winnicott, 1964/1992). Conversely, if early attachment relationships are neglectful or hurtful, children are likely to approach future relationships with wariness or profound neediness (Bowlby, 1969; Brown & Elliott, 2016; Schore, 2001, 2015; Tronick, 2007).

A good understanding of attachment disruption is foundational for family therapists, as even minor attachment disruptions can have global, lifelong, and intergenerational impact. It is our job to bring prevention and repair to our clients, and prevention and repair are possible. This section lays out preventative strategies—those that will transform the attachment environment of children's homes, preventing attachment disruption. It also describes healing strategies for when things have already gone awry. Even in an environment where past hurts and losses have already had a negative impact, attuned, warm parents with adequate knowledge can create a healing climate. There is always a reason for hope.

FOSTERING SECURITY WITH PARENTS FIRST: ATTUNE, INFORM, AND STRATEGIZE

In treatment, positive energy and resources flow downhill from provider to parent and parent to child. When a child shows up for treatment, the initial job of providers is to begin building an attuned relationship with the parent and to instill hope in the parent that healing is possible. To this end, we recommend therapists begin treatment with a focus on:

1. Developing an emotional bond with the parent.
2. Providing an understandable explanation of the presenting concern.
3. Formulating a realistic plan for healing that is accepted by the parent.
4. Establishing a process through which healing can begin.

Communicate hope and optimism. Your knowledge and confidence will increase your persuasiveness and the client's trust and willingness to engage (Laska et al., 2014; Wampold, 2017). An attuned therapeutic relationship like this one will immediately reduce parental stress in the home. Collaborative family work will lower the risks of children's mistreatment or neglect (Baylin & Hughes, 2016; Burke, 2010; Chen et al., 2018; Davidson & McEwen, 2012; Dobbs, 2009; Heinicke et al., 1999; Hoffman et al., 2006; Juffer et al., 2017; Bakermans-Kranenburg et al., 2005).

SECURE FOUNDATION

Intimate relational experiences in the early years of life shape children's developing sense of self, relational abilities, and overall confidence. Early feelings of pride or shame, acceptance or rejection, begin to form children's sense of their place in the world. Healthy social and emotional development depends on having at least one attentive, responsive adult with whom to interact. Without a responsive caretaker, children's social abilities are more likely to be impaired (Bowlby, 1952, 1969; Brazelton & Greenspan, 2001; Brown & Elliott, 2016; Cozolino, 2014; Lester & Sparrow, 2010; Medina, 2014; Schore, 2012, 2017).

It is within a steady, healthy parent–child relationship that children can build a solid sense of security. The parents' ability to enjoy and appreciate them, respond to their feelings and needs, and comfort them in troubled times are the raw materials of attachment security. When these are present, children are set up to build self-confidence, emotional awareness, positive social behavior, and trust.

When parents are supportive, protective, and reliable, children feel secure and can thrive. The repeated experience of being seen, understood, and well-paced creates in children a sense of safety and of being valued. Such experiences demonstrate to children that their thoughts and feelings are legitimate and make sense, leading children to a deep understanding and acceptance of themselves and their perceptions. Their later emotions, behaviors, and experiences are all colored by this early-established sense of self. Children can then pass forward their emotional sensitivity and caring to their peers in the future. This dynamic process is the result of a secure attachment.

The view of themselves and the world that is formed by early attachment experiences is literally encoded in children's developing brains. When children are met with a hopeful stance, they are led to recreate positivity and success. Positive attachments lay a sound foundation for relational trust and prosocial behavior (Bowlby, 1969; Cassidy et al., 2013; Fonagy et al., 2010; Karen, 1998; Schore, 2012; Siegel, 2020; Tronick, 2007; Winnicott, 1964/1992).

Secure and reliable early connections create expectations for trust and collaboration with others. They also set children up to be sensitive to others, read social cues, and have sound social judgment. Such relational experiences can lead to self-fulfilling prophecies—a positive feedback cycle—as new people in children's lives tend to mirror their friendliness or distance. Children with positive connections will appear more open and warm, which makes it easier for them to create new friendships. On the other hand, if children's early attachments are insecure or hurtful, they are set up for negative expectations in relationships. These children may appear overly anxious or distant from others, which can interfere with building new connections and reinforce social insecurities (Brazelton & Greenspan, 2001; Cozolino, 2014; Main & Hesse, 1990).

According to *World Happiness Report 2017*, a robust social foundation ("having someone to count on") is the single most potent factor related to happiness in life evaluations across countries—stronger than health and income (Helliwell et al., 2017). Bowlby saw this clearly in 1952, when he wrote for the World Health Organization that it is "believed to be essential for mental health that the infant and young child should experience warm, intimate, and continuous relationship with its mother (or permanent mother substitute) in which both find satisfaction and enjoyment."

PROGRESSION OF EARLY ATTACHMENT AND SOCIAL–EMOTIONAL CAPACITIES

In the first few weeks of life, an infant begins to interact with the world and to manage states of mind between wakefulness and sleep. After a few weeks, infants can recognize and seek out primary caregivers. Early nonverbal and automatic imitation of caregiver behavior, such as tongue protrusion, mouth opening, and smiling, facilitates early bonding within hours of birth. Parents promote the infant's social development by responding to these early signals. Ideal responses are at a matched pace and meet the infant's need for interaction, novelty, and attachment.

In the following months, the baby begins to exchange more intentional facial expressions and vocal sounds with parents. Early cooing and gestures are the start of their social engagement. Between the ages of 2 and 4 months, the baby will start to discriminate between caregivers. They can show a clear preference for primary caregivers by the age of 3 months, orienting to and greeting parents and beginning to play with pace and rhythm in relational exchanges. Within this developmental stage, the full range of basic emotions can be experienced. Around 4 months, children will have developed the beginnings of internal behavioral control, allowing them to take the lead in interactions and playing social games.

Between 4 and 6 months, babies are forming inner feelings of trust and security. Social interactions between parents and children become more intentional and collaborative. Around 6 to 9 months, children become aware of being separate from caregivers. A healthy identity arises from early foundations of being appreciated and seen as a separate individual in their relationship with caregivers. They also begin to feel more wary of unknown adults (stranger anxiety), as their new cognitive skill of person permanence allows them to realize some adults are not their caregivers.

Through the ninth to 12th months of life, children's growing cognitive and emotional capacities will allow for the discrimination of different emotional experiences. Emotions can become more complex and less automatic in experience and expression. Parents can assist in deepening emotional awareness and regulation through reflecting and articulating children's feelings, remaining attuned, and providing appropriate soothing.

By around 18 months, children have developed the capacity for representational and symbolic thinking, which allows for a maturing sense of self. They can discriminate more clearly between themselves and others. Children of this age are more sophisticated at reading nonverbal cues such as body language and facial expressions, and begin to use simple words to communicate, such as "more," "bye-bye," and "mama." They begin to substitute words or body language to express thoughts and feelings rather than automatic behaviors. Newly mature verbal and nonverbal skills replace more immature behavioral reactions.

By the age of 2 years, most children have developed a clear internal representation of self and others. Between 2 and 4 years, as cognitive sophistication grows, children begin to articulate thoughts, feelings, and intentions. At this stage, they can verbally protest an experience that does not match their desire. This is why 2-year-olds say "no." They can also use their expanding vocabulary to represent feelings and behaviors. Symbolic play—playing pretend with others—begins during this stage.

In the first few years, children's unique patterns of managing inner thoughts and feelings, coping with stress, and interacting with others are already being formed. At each of the stages described below, caregivers have a unique and timely window to help shape children's sense of self and others (Table 3.1). As a therapist, recognizing the appropriate parental role in facilitating good attachment throughout early life will support you in guiding, course correcting, and developing healing strategies for clients and families.

Table 3.1 PROGRESSING ATTACHMENT INTERACTIONS: CHILD SOCIAL DEVELOPMENT AND PARENTAL ROLES		
Age	Child's Developing Social Behavior	Developing Parental Role
1–3 weeks	Reflexive facial mimicry, emerging attachment interactions, maintaining alert states	Eye contact and interaction, balancing engagement and rest
3–8 weeks	Identify primary caregivers, cooing, intentional facial expressions, gestures	Exchange vocal and facial expressions
2–3 months	Preference for primary caregivers, begin playful interchanges with adults, begin to experience full range of emotions, less reflexive and more intentional behavior	Simple, playful exchanges with rhythm and reciprocity with primary caregivers, acknowledge and respond to a full range of emotions with compassion
3–4 months	Forming independence, control, or leading adults in simple play, self-soothing to rest and stay attentive to exciting situations	Respect and facilitate baby's shifts in interactions or play; support self-regulation when accessible to the baby, offer new experiences when alert
4–6 months	Building inner security, learning to trust and seek connections, reciprocal play with facial expressions	Mutually dramatic play, positive interactions, enhance fun and joy in interactions
6–9 months	Sense of self, awareness of caregivers versus strangers	Pride in the child's sense of self, attentive, encouraging, attuned, and playful, emotionally sensitive to stranger anxiety
9–12 months	Stabilize attachment patterns, differentiate emotions	Mirror and soothe emotions, assist with self-regulation

12–18 months	Early sense of self, stable attachment patterns, learn to read and use nonverbal cues such as body language and facial expressions	Appreciation of child's budding self, loving verbal interactions and play, responsive to child's behavioral experimentation
18–24 months	Internalized attachment patterns, stronger internal models of self and others, identity formation	Reflection of a valued and unique self, deepening cocreated attachment patterns, a secure base from which to self-soothe and explore new situations and people
2–4 years	Stable internal representations of attachment, self, and others, substitute a thought for an action, mental images can represent needs and emotions, symbolic play	Talk about feelings and behavior, encourage early use of emotional expression, set limits while nurturing autonomy, sensitivity to a new sense of self and potential feelings of shame

SOURCE: Brazelton & Greenspan, 2001; Brazelton & Sparrow, 2006; Brown & Elliott, 2016.

NEUROBIOLOGY OF ATTACHMENT: BORN TO ATTACH

Babies become familiar with caretakers before they are aware of their own existence. Even during pregnancy, the baby starts to develop connections to the mother and other family members.

Physical regulation of the body and mind begins before birth, in utero, and is strongly influenced by maternal physical and emotional state. The fetus moves, shifts, changes states of alertness and adjusts its heart rate in response to the mother. Even the stress level of a mother during pregnancy has an impact on the fetus; lasting impact can be seen in the child's reactions to stress during the first months of life (Huizink et al., 2003; Lester & Sparrow, 2010; Schetter & Tanner, 2012).

As evidenced by infants' reactions after birth to voices they heard while in utero, a fetus can hear voices from the outer world during later pregnancy. Talking or singing to the baby during pregnancy is one way that mothers, fathers, and siblings can start to form connections with that baby before birth. In the first hours of life, most babies start to respond to the people around them. They are not the passive recipients of attention we once thought. Babies can begin to smile and mimic behavior from day one (Brazelton & Sparrow, 2006; Medina, 2014). By nature, we crave intimate connection with others. This is a primary drive already in place at birth. The complexity of the social dance gets more sophisticated over the early months as neurons fire and form new connections.

In the first year of life, babies are sensitive to the tone, rhythm, and pacing of interactions, which are processed primarily by the right side of the brain. At that time, the right hemisphere is dominant and is growing faster than the left (Medina, 2014; Schore, 2001, 2015). As presented in Chapter 2, the right hemisphere helps us with facial recognition, spatial ability, and visual imagery. The left hemisphere—more logical, linear, and language focused—grows more slowly in the first year of life, becoming dominant around the fourth year. It is during these early years that children lay the groundwork for future ability to read others and connect to them in nonverbal ways. This development is the foundation of attachment.

Our brains possess mirror neurons that foster attachment. They promote attunement by allowing us to feel one another's intent or emotions at a physiological level. When we watch someone move their body with intention—kicking a ball, for example, or eating a sandwich—our mirror neurons can be triggered (Iacoboni, 2009). In our own bodies, similar neurological signals are sent without the associated muscle movement. Mirror neurons are at the root of our ability to feel sad in the face of another's pain or excited for another's success. Our brains pick up the cues on another person's face in 100 milliseconds. In 300 milliseconds, the muscles in our faces may already mirror what we notice on the other person's face (Panksepp & Biven, 2012). All of this happens outside of our conscious awareness. This neurobiological response sets the stage for parents to smoothly respond to infants' oscillating needs for safety and connection, stimulation, soothing, or exploration.

Attachment is such a prerequisite for healthy growth that children do not develop well emotionally, cognitively, or physically if attachment relationships are gravely disrupted. Sound relational support in childhood shapes the brain and body in broad and long-lasting ways.

SIBLING ATTACHMENT IN TWINS

Twin children have the good fortune to have an additional primary attachment: each other. Children commonly bond with siblings, but usually only form attachment relationships with one or two primary adult caretakers. Twins, however, often form close attachment connections with each other. The twin cannot replace the primary adult attachment, but it is another significant source of love and support for them.

When my twin sons were about 15 months old, they began day care for the first time. By this age, they were tightly bonded with both parents, their nanny, and each other. During one of their first days in out-of-home care, they went out to play on the playground with their class. Playtime ended, and their teacher called for them to come to the gate to head back to class.

The older twin heard, understood, and cooperatively went to join his teacher at the gate. He soon noticed his brother was still playing. He panicked, ran to his brother, grabbed him by the head, and tried to drag him to the gate. At this young age, he was already attentive to and connected with his brother. He felt separation stress and concern for maintaining proximity, and took responsibility to be sure both were well.

E. S.

ATTACHMENT IN THE ANIMAL WORLD

Attachment security is a requirement for healthy development—and not just for humans. It is also true for much of the animal world. Phyllis Lee from the University of Stirling found that elephants with an attentive maternal figure in the first five years of life were more likely to survive and reproduce. When a supportive mother figure was not present, the young elephants were less likely to reach full growth size and more likely to die young. Males were more vulnerable than females to the costs of not having a caring maternal caretaker. It was found that the adverse effects of having an inexperienced or absent maternal figure could be buffered by having an older maternal advocate in the group or a particularly positive adult elephant community (Kinver, 2013; Lee et al., 2013).

Similarly, research with our near cousin, the rhesus monkey, has shown that regardless of the baby monkey's innate disposition (sturdy, rough, or sensitive), the temperament and caregiving style of the mother monkey strongly predicts the baby's future survival and social and reproductive success. Especially nurturing mothers produced normally functioning monkeys, even when the baby was nervous to begin with. Abusive mothers produced very anxious monkeys (Dobbs, 2009; Suomi, 2005).

Even a rat benefits from a close and comforting relationship with its mother. Research has found that rat pups whose mothers responded to stress by licking and grooming them grew larger, were less anxious and less aggressive, and were more social, curious, intelligent, and healthier than those whose dams were less nurturing (Todeschin et al., 2009). Even more impressive, further research demonstrated that rat pups with highly nurturing dams not only had demonstrably different concentrations of neurotransmitters than pups who received less licking and grooming; greater nurturing was also correlated with differences in DNA. A part of the genome responsible for managing stress was activated in the pups of more affectionate dams (Caldji et al., 2000).

PARENT–CHILD ATTACHMENT CATEGORIES

We have thoroughly described ideal conditions for secure, healthy parent–child attachment to foster optimal mental, physical, social, and psychological well-being. Now, we'll look at the patterns of behavior that are most likely to arise in children who are securely attached—as well as those that suggest insecure or disorganized attachment.

Social scientists have studied attachment categories for decades. Through this research, scientists have grouped children's attachment relationship with their parent into four distinct categories: secure, insecure ambivalent, insecure avoidant, and disorganized (Bowlby, 1969; Karen, 1998; Main, 2006; Schore, 2015; Tronick, 2007; Wallin, 2007; Winnicott, 1964/1992). These four attachment categories are seen across cultures.

In 1970, Mary Ainsworth created the Infant Strange Situation to study different types of attachment between mothers and babies (Ainsworth et al., 1978). As a result of that research, the first three types of attachment were identified. In later years, Mary Main's research on attachment added the fourth category of attachment—disorganized or disoriented—to the literature (Main & Solomon, 1990).

The Infant Strange Situation test involves placing a mother and young child (1 to 2 years old) in a room with toys and an observer who is a stranger to the child. After the mother gets the child acclimated, she leaves the room temporarily. Observations of the child's reactions when the mother returns yield information about how that child is attached.

Secure Attachment

Secure parent–child attachments are seen in homes with caretakers who are safe, caring, available, and predictable. Children in secure homes tend to feel understood and cared about there; they know they are accepted as they are and feel free to know and express their feelings. Securely attached children are allowed to feel free and valuable in the world. Guiding, protective limits are set and held by caretakers.

Secure homes are often run by parents who were raised securely themselves. Even with no parental training, they naturally raise secure children. This pattern is documented in the research; parental attachment status influences the parent–child attachment relationship via the parents' emotional and relational capacities. Research indicates that secure attachment categories are found in slightly over half of all people (Bakermans-Kranenburg & van IJzendoorn, 2009). This percentage appears to have declined in the past few decades, as security was found to be present in two-thirds of attachments a few decades ago. This change suggests that society may be moving in a less emotionally connected direction (Moullin et al., 2018).

In the Strange Situation, securely attached children are upset by separation from the mother, but are quick to recover, seek connection, and get back to play after she returns.

Insecure Attachment

Children are more likely to develop insecure attachment relationships when raised in homes where parents are less reliable and struggle with their own emotional lives. In the case of ambivalent insecure parent–child attachments, parents tend to be preoccupied by their own trauma or loss, easily angered, and can shift between being intrusive or withdrawn in relationship with their children. They are more likely to be misattuned, inconsistently available, and confusing to children. In *avoidant insecure* parent–child attachments, parents are likely to be emotionally detached in interactions, unavailable, or dismissive of emotions. They are more distant, less caring, and lacking in emotional attunement. An increase in the avoidant attachment category is found in more recent research (Konrath et al., 2014).

It is important to note that even secure homes have moments of insecurity. There are degrees of insecurity and chaos in all homes, and this does not preclude secure attachment in the presence of overall security or good-enough parenting. No parent is perfect.

In the Strange Situation, when the parent–child attachment status is ambivalent insecure, children are often distressed prior to the separation and are not easily soothed after the mother's return. They do not return to playfulness. When the parent–child attachment status is avoidant insecure, children do not show behavioral signs of distress and continue to play, even with the stranger— although physiological measures indicate an intense internal stress reaction.

Disorganized Attachment

When the home environment produces a deeply conflicting urge in the child to go to the caretaker for security, but also flee the caretaker as a source of fear or instability, a disorganized attachment strategy can form in the parent–child relationship. In these relationships the child feels grave instability as they experience the parent as frightening, frightened, disoriented, or terrifying. There is no ready strategy or solution for children in this extreme stress. They may cope through dissociation, or develop a fragmented sense of self, and an erratic way of relating to others (Ainsworth et al., 1978; Schore, 2015; Main & Hesse, 1990). Although childhood abuse can result in disorganized attachment, abuse is not always present.

In the Strange Situation, when the parent–child attachment status is disorganzied, children respond to their caregiver in unusual ways prior to the separation. Upon reunion, their behavior remains disorganized or disoriented, reflecting the absence of an organized attachment strategy. They may wander, freeze in place, or engage in undirected movement. Their behavior is considered by researchers to display "fright without a solution" (Main & Hesse, 1990; Siegel, 2020).

Attachment Categories at a Birthday Party

While the parent–child attachment status is predictive of the ways in which a child will behave in relationships, it also reflects how the parent is likely to behave—and has probably behaved as a general rule—in the parent–child dynamic (see Table 3.2). On the other hand, parents' attachment histories alone do not accurately predict their ability to create a secure parent–child relationship, rather it is parents' understanding and integration of their own histories that determines whether they can create an attuned and secure connection for their children. Parents who have worked through insecure or painful histories with a process of self-reflection, can then create sensitive and reliable attachment relationships with their children. The parent's work on themselves provides them with a healthier attachment pattern called "earned security," discussed further in Chapter 6 (Siegel, 2020).

Here we will explore how different attachment strategies might look in a similar scenario: a birthday party. Imagine a child excitedly preparing for his third birthday party. Just before guests arrive, he puts his fingers into the cake sitting on the counter. Most parents would feel upset or flustered, but their responses would vary greatly depending on their attachment strategy.

A parent with a secure attachment pattern would recover more quickly from being upset than other attachment patterns. They might accept the child's excited feelings about the cake, fix the cake, explain to the child the limits with the cake, and get ready for the party, with the cake now out of the child's reach.

A parent with an ambivalent insecure attachment pattern would be more easily triggered by their emotions and might respond with quick, intense anger, followed by feelings of guilt or remorse. They may cater to their child apologetically and be slow to recover emotionally. The child would be likely to feel confused or worried by the parent's anger and sadness; the parental tension would transmit to the child.

A parent with an avoidant insecure attachment pattern would be more likely to be dismissive. They may be coldly angry or disinterested in whether or not the child is touching the cake. The avoidant parent primarily operates from their own needs and is less likely than the other styles to talk with the child about what happened. This parent may not appear upset, but their body would be tense and slow to recover.

A parent with a disorganized attachment pattern may be aggressive with the child, irrationally enraged, or may appear overwhelmed entirely by the issue and burst into childish tears. The child is left feeling fearful and with a sense that things are out of control, with no resources for recovery or comfort in the parent. In this example, we can observe how these experiences, when repeated over time, can shape children's expectations and reactions in the larger world.

Table 3.2 SUMMARY OF ATTACHMENT CATEGORIES AND ASSOCIATED PARENTING BEHAVIORS	
Parent–Child Attachment	**Parenting Patterns Observed**
Secure	Emotionally and physically available, reliable, and responsive
Ambivalent Insecure	Preoccupied with their internal experiences, irritable, intrusive, and inconsistent
Avoidant Insecure	Unavailable, neglectful, unaware, or rejecting
Disorganized	Frightened, terrifying, disorienting, or dysregulated

RANGES OF ATTACHMENT SECURITY

Many shades of security can exist between safe and unsafe. Some families hold some aspects of security and lack others. For example, a stoic parent may offer physical protection, material goods, and supervision, but lack emotional connection, or a sense of caring genuinely at an emotional level. Or a family may accept positive feelings, but not allow the expression of any negative affect such as anger or sadness. This pattern can cause the child to be strong in some areas while lacking in others. Also, it only allows for partial integration rather than a full acceptance of the self with all the good and bad emotions that come with it.

When a child has a mix of primary relationship experiences, they can have a blended parent–child attachment strategy. One parent may create a secure connection while the other is very insecure in their interactions with the child. This discrepancy can create a combination of expectations for the child or a blended parent–child attachment status that shifts based on the environment.

The parent–child attachment foundation plays a major role in building our neurobiological foundation. This being said, also know that early attachment patterns are not locked in. Neuroplasticity indicates that change can occur later in life. The amount of change possible may be dependent on the age of intervention, opportunities for secure connection, and support for repair and emotional integration of past adversity (Cramer et al., 2011; Davidson & McEwen, 2012; Lester & Sparrow, 2010; Siegel, 2020; Vance et al., 2010).

Parents' abilities to meet their children's connection needs are heavily influenced by the parents' own attachment strategy. Parents with secure histories, or those who have worked to understand and integrate their insecure histories, will find it easier to attune to and sensitively care for their children in a good-enough way. However, parents with their unaddressed attachment insecurity may have difficulty pacing, regulating, and sensitively attending to their children (Ainsworth et al., 1978; Ainsworth & Eichberg, 2006; Karen, 1998; Main, 2006; Main & Hesse, 1990; Siegel, 2020; Winnicott, 1964/1992). As a result, the parents' connections with their children are heavily influenced by the parents' ability to be available for secure attachment, and this can lead to the perpetuation of the parents' attachment patterns. In other words, the parent's current state of mind regarding their attachment strategy can be transmitted intergenerationally.

Although attachment strategies tend to be passed down from parent to child, significant changes in a child's life, such as loss, can alter feelings of security. The sudden loss of a positive attachment figure or significant trauma can introduce anxiety and can also trigger feelings of grief and depression (Bowlby, 1969; Ainsworth & Eichberg, 2006; Tronick, 2007, 2017; Waters et al., 2000). On the other hand, the introduction of a new secure attachment can bring a stronger sense of safety to a person with an unsafe history. While our expectations of social safety are built by early experience, later experiences can change expectations.

4

Ideal Scenarios: Building Family Security and Positive Identity

Emotional and physical health develop naturally for children under the right conditions. There is a finite set of essential childhood needs that, when met, create the proper conditions for sound development. Paramount among these is a stable and secure parent–child attachment (Bowlby, 1969; Brazelton & Greenspan, 2001; Brazelton & Sparrow, 2006; Brown & Elliott, 2016; Cozolino, 2014; Karen, 1998; Lester & Sparrow, 2010; Schore, 2012, 2017; Tronick, 2007; Winnicott, 1964/1992).

In the first part of this book, we reviewed developmental theory and psychological research, and we integrated our own clinical experience to formulate a list of 7 essential attachment needs for healthy attachment. When these needs are met, they offer children an optimal environment in which to grow and thrive.

THE 7 ESSENTIAL ATTACHMENT NEEDS

Essential attachment need #1: safety and security. By offering safety and security, parents create an environment where children learn that their family is a safe place, and then naturally develop a foundation of trust in the world.

Children who feel safe and secure at home learn that they can count on being sheltered from danger and that they are loved and worthy of being protected and cared for.

Essential attachment need #2: soothing. Next, physical and emotional soothing from parents during moments of struggle creates the conditions for childhood resilience, building trust on the part of children that their parents can buffer stressful circumstances. Eventually, after many iterations of being soothed, children become familiar with the cycle of stress, soothing, and relief; this is how they learn to self-soothe. Resilience grows from a deep understanding that misery will pass and that one is capable of recovery. Being comforted by parents also lays the foundation for emotional awareness and self-regulation later in life (Blair, 2008; Brody et al., 2010; Hackman et al., 2013; Tronick, 2007; Vandell, 2010) and reinforces the message to the child that they are worthy of care.

Essential attachment need #3: attunement. Another essential dimension of a nurturing parent–child relationship is attunement. This quality develops when parents tune in to their children's experiences and show resonant compassion for them. Attunement offers the experience of being seen and valued by an important other. Emotional attunement implicitly validates children's needs and feelings, communicating that they are acceptable and legitimate. Over time, children who receive attunement are able to offer attunement to others. Their expression of empathy for others can result in the formation of positive, healthy relationships.

Essential attachment need #4: reliability and consistency. When parents are reliable and consistent, children can develop full trust in the relationship. They know their parents are there and can be counted on. They are not confused; they know what is going to happen and how parents will respond, which promotes a feeling of calm. Reliable adults also provide a model for children on how to live with discipline and responsibility.

Essential attachment need #5: support and encouragement. Children also need emotional support and encouragement. By showing faith in the child, the adult supports them to see themselves in a positive light even when circumstances are difficult. Receiving the gift of time and effort from significant adults once again communicates that the child is valuable, interesting, and worthy.

Essential attachment need #6: play and fun. Let's not forget about play and fun (stimulation, novelty, and pleasure), which are hugely attractive to children and invigorating for all of us. Meeting these needs helps build a pleasurable bond between parents and children. An atmosphere of play and fun also offers a place for children to develop familiarity with positive emotions and the ability to create positivity in their lives.

Essential attachment need #7: boundaries and structure. All of this growth and excitement must be balanced with clear family rules, schedules, and expectations, which create a sense of security and confidence. As children predictably know what is going to happen—what is in and out of bounds—they gradually grow confident they can function within expectations. Setting limits with children is critical for keeping chaos out of the family and fostering stability, self-efficacy, and self-control. It also sets the stage for children learning to set boundaries with others and to understand that limit setting is a normal part of life.

When parents can meet children's essential attachment needs, their children feel held and nurtured in the relationship. This is secure attachment. But it is not an all-or-nothing formula. All parents have strengths in certain areas and find others harder to provide consistently. As therapists, our goal is to recognize the importance of all of these areas; to identify those that could use some bolstering; and to work with parents to support them in doing just that. Research has documented again and again that secure attachment is indeed a prerequisite for optimal emotional, relational, and behavioral functioning (Ainsworth et al., 1978; Baylin & Hughes, 2016; Bowlby, 1952, 1969; Cozolino, 2014; Fonagy et al., 2010; Karen, 1998; Main, 1990, 2006; Porges, 2011; Schore, 2015; Siegel, 2017; Tronick, 2007, 2017; Waters et al., 2000; Winnicott, 1964/1992).

ATTUNEMENT: QUALITY OF CONNECTION

Among the 7 essential attachment needs, attunement stands out as a necessary component for most of the others. The quality of attunement in the parent–child connection has far-reaching effects on children's daily experiences. In attuned relationships, children feel seen and are reliably granted their parents' steadying connection. Attuned parents anchor their children. Attunement provides validation of children's core worth. It is within these attuned relationships that people can feel deep intimacy and love.

When parents attune with their children, they allow their physical and mental states to shift to join with or balance those of their children. When parents are attentive and appropriately responsive to children's feelings and thoughts, the parent–child connection is an attuned one, and the members of the dyad feel closely connected. This closeness, which involves parents being mindful to sense and reflect children's state of mind, can be accomplished with body language, touch, or words demonstrating the parents' accurate responsiveness to the child's emotional states. This ensures that the child feels understood and valued, which is at the heart of building a secure relationship (Baylin & Hughes, 2016; Cozolino, 2014; Field, 2014; Gross, 2014; Heller, 1997; Lester & Sparrow, 2010; Schore, 2012, Siegel 2020).

In the first few years, caregivers attune by responding to children's cues. Some cues are dramatic and undeniable, as when infants are screaming and red-faced. However, attuned parents also take note of the subtleties of children's early efforts to communicate. For example, a child turning toward a parent can suggest readiness for interaction or play, while fussing or turning away can indicate a need for quiet or rest. As children mature, these expressions continue, but in the familiarity of the parent–child dance, they are more readily decoded and attuned to. Attuned parents are able to notice what children need, and also when their current need has been met.

Through experiencing attunement, children learn to recognize, express, and honor their own emotional lives—a set of abilities that lie at the core of self-worth. Being accurately mirrored helps children see themselves and grow in the belief that they are worthy of having their needs met and of being respected by others. As children receive empathy, they develop the capacity to have compassion for others. This type of connection is essential to prepare children to develop long-term intimate relationships later in life.

Parents cannot attune to children all of the time. Fortunately, constant attunement is not needed to create attachment security. It is not natural for someone to be always in sync with another person; parents and children are individuals and need space for their individual needs. Instead, the parent–child relationship is a fluid dance of connection, distance, and reconnecting. What matters is that children experience this attuned connection on a regular enough basis and know that it is accessible in times of need. Parents who can attune to their children find the other essential attachment needs easier to meet and can meet them more smoothly.

TRUST: CONNECTED RESPONSIVENESS

Most babies enter the world primed to connect with others. They give their parents cues about what they want and need, and take in information from their parents. Eventually, children learn to trust others if their parents are sensitive to and reliably meet their needs, and if those parents are emotionally steady. This type of connected responsiveness can include parents showing interest and pleasure in children, adjusting play to what they enjoy, and accommodating their preferences when possible, articulating children's feelings, acknowledging their reactions, and adjusting to their rhythms.

No specific parent behavior guarantees adequate building of trust; rather, parents' appropriate responsiveness to the child's shifting needs is what contributes most. When parents attend to their children, not just words and cries, but their facial expressions, body language, tone of voice, and pacing, the parents gather information that will allow them to meet their needs. This process can feel like parental intuition, or it can be consciously observed and considered.

Of course, this is more easily accomplished when children and parents are both in positive moods and moving at a similar pace. When the child or parent is upset, this connected responsiveness is both more challenging and more important. Attempting to stay lovingly connected and succeeding during hard times—at least somewhat—helps the child learn to trust. During these times of upset, attachment-aware parents recognize the importance of not overreacting or underreacting. Tuning into children's experiences in a caring way when they are upset, and accepting and respecting their feelings is a tremendous support for trusting attachment.

When children are upset, parents can tune in to the children's experiences and accept and respect their feelings. When parents are upset, it is incumbent on them to manage their own emotions and not take them out on the child. This self-regulation creates emotional safety for the child and the awareness that negative feelings are normal and can be tolerated by parents. It leads to the sense that the world and others are safe, that it is safe to try new things, and that having a feeling or making a mistake is not beyond repair.

An interesting phenomenon often occurs as parents read their children's frame of mind and react accordingly: Children begin to read their parents' frames of mind and to respond to them. They start to see their parents as individuals and to take cues from them. This is visible in infancy, continues to develop across childhood, and is fostered within ongoing, positively attuned parent–child relationships. In the process of this trusting dance of reading and responding to one another, mutual bonding occurs and is reinforced. These relationships are trust-based secure attachments.

BODY LANGUAGE AND CONNECTION

In the ideal attachment scenario, parents' interactions with their children are congruent, both verbally and nonverbally. Efforts at attunement are read as authentic when the more subtle nonverbal cues of interest and concern are consistent with the parent's actions and words. Such authenticity strengthens attachment security.

Authentic interaction feels honest and sincere, not fabricated or shallow. Resonant connection holds the quality of harmony and understanding between people. The relationship flows and makes sense. In a congruent interaction, verbal and nonverbal expressions are harmonious with one another. When a person's communication is congruent, they come across as thoughtful and honest (Cozolino, 2014; Siegel, 2020).

Aware parents are conscious of their nonverbal communication and work to align their verbal and nonverbal expressions. For example, at the end of a long day, parents' way of greeting their children communicates information about their feelings toward them, whether they intend it to or not. Parents wanting to show happiness upon seeing their children are undermined in doing so if their nonverbal gestures and facial expressions fail to reflect their pleasure. A calm smile would be registered as warm and caring, while a neutral, tense, or negative face could be interpreted as detached or rejecting, even if the accompanying words are warm.

Body cues are registered immediately, without conscious awareness. We automatically respond to others' posture, facial expressions, and gestures. The right side of our brain readily picks up nonverbal signals and prepares us to respond. When words are consistent with body language, the interaction is coherent. If body language is inconsistent, the resulting confusion interferes with connection.

Our natural ability to read a person's nonverbal communication is at the root of our capacity to tell a lie from the truth, a manipulation from an honest action, or a surface compliment from genuine appreciation. When you have an intuitive feeling that someone is not telling the truth, it is often because your right hemisphere is picking up the incongruence between the spoken and unspoken words. Children have this intuitive ability from early on. When a parent's behavior is incongruent, the child is likely to notice and feel confused and torn. They have to choose between trusting the parent's word and trusting themselves.

POSITIVE SELF-IMAGE: DEVELOPS IN CONNECTION

When things go well with the parent–child attachment relationship, positive identity is a predictable outcome. Children develop their self-image, which is their story about themselves, from their experiences and the feedback they receive from the people around them. All of the narrative bits of knowledge and suppositions about the self come together to form an identity—a sense of self created across the course of a lifetime. How children are spoken to and treated by their primary caretakers lays the groundwork for their identity.

The story, or narrative, is both explicit and implicit. Children can overtly think and feel, "I am loveable. I am strong. I am happy" or "I am weak. I am insignificant. I am unlovable." These self-views can also be implicit, such as when children have a feeling of confidence or a vague sense of worthlessness without knowing why. Their beliefs and narratives can be in awareness or below awareness.

Narratives: Explicit and Implicit Memory

Memories preserve our experiences; narratives help us make sense of our memories. Memories are explicit and implicit—they influence both our stories about ourselves. Explicit memories, when recalled, are linked to past events (such as episodic, semantic, and autobiographical memories). They feel like a recollection of an event. Implicit memories, when recalled, are not experienced as linked to the past—rather they are experienced as true in the moment (such as procedural, priming, or conditioned memories). They are experienced as a known skill, an accepted bit of understanding, or even a flashback. Both types of memory influence our daily experiences and our conceptualizations about ourselves.

These types of memory are stored in the brain in different ways. Explicit memories are processed by the hippocampus (for higher brain and cortical learning). Implicit memories are processed without hippocampal involvement, they involve primarily limbic regions, amygdala and other subcortical regions, and motor areas. Implicit memories can prepare the brain to respond in certain ways by creating mental models or schema across experiences (Cozolino, 2014; Dubuc, 2013; Siegel, 2020).

Explicit memories can be recalled as part of the past. They can be about personal experiences (for example, a trip you took two years ago), something learned (for example, knowledge of the events leading up to the Civil War), or something experienced in the world (the events of 9/11). *Implicit memories*, although not having the internal sensation of being linked to past experiences, are stored in our neurobiology and can influence our behaviors and emotions. Examples of implicit memory in action include how to drive a car, type on a keyboard, navigate a familiar neighborhood, or sing a familiar song.

These different types of memories are stored in different parts of the brain. Explicit memory is stored in the hippocampus and prefrontal cortex, while implicit memory is stored in the amygdala (Cozolino, 2014; Dubuc, 2013; Siegel, 2020).

These memories from narratives about the self create a mental expectation, which can become a self-fulfilling prophecy. For example, when children feel valuable and confident, they approach life with enthusiasm and resilience that can build on itself. They are game in the face of challenges. Their assurance plays out in repeated experiences of fun and accomplishment, as well as in success navigating failures. These then further fuel their positive self-image. A child who feels insignificant and unlovable is likely to have very different experiences because of the way the child shows up in interactions.

This type of experience can run across all facets of one's identity. If a child thinks he is good at learning, he will approach his assignments with confidence. He will be thorough, willing to ask questions, and likely to remember to turn in his work. All of this increases the positive feedback the child receives from his parents and teachers and the likelihood of good grades, further increasing his confidence. Similarly, if a child thinks he is bad at soccer, he will approach practice with trepidation, cut corners to hide his incompetence, feel afraid to ask for coaching, and prefer to sit on the bench. All of these increase the negative feedback the child receives from coaches, team members, and parents, further decreasing his confidence.

CONNECTING AROUND SUCCESS

Children develop a positive sense of self when they have experiences of success and can take in that success. Parents cannot create those experiences for them; they must be created by the children. Parents can, however, work to be sure children are aware of and can absorb successes as they happen. Within the context of the attachment relationship, parents authentically lighting up with pride and speaking of children's successes provide powerful encouragement to children to take note of the truth of their accomplishments. This positive cycle occurs often and naturally when things are going well in the relationship.

Children do not feel a strong sense of success and pride when feedback is a muted "Good job!" or "Here, take this trophy." Children crave and benefit from more detailed, accurate recognition that is specific to them. It feels nourishing to hear, "You have a very good mind for basketball. You are always in the right place at the right time. You anticipate the next play quite well." When this type of feedback is accurate, it resonates as valid for the child, which builds positive self-knowledge. It allows them to clarify their identity as someone with a good mind and who has the gift of anticipation.

Inaccurate feedback, even if positive, is not powerful. Take, for example, the not-uncommon practice of awarding every child a trophy at the end of a sports season. Trophies given by default do not provide accurate feedback about children's skills and accomplishments. They are, rather, tokens of participation and community. Children know this and value them as such.

DEVELOPMENTAL PROGRESSION OF IDENTITY

Children's sense of self develops within their attachment relationships and in response to experience and feedback from the world. The developmental and biological substrate on which identity is built moves through a progression of steps. Just as there are stages in attachment development, there are stages in identity development. Identity is essentially cocreated by children and the central people in their lives across these stages.

Even tiny babies take in information from the world about themselves, but they do not take it in via language as do older children. Here are some general guidelines for understanding the development of positive identity and sense of self—and parental role in supporting this development—throughout childhood and into early adulthood.

In the first year of life, babies' identities are created within the relationship with their primary caretakers. In the first few months, an infant cannot yet hold a separate, concrete sense of self. A baby's identity starts with physical body awareness and starts to include emotions and traits such as likes and dislikes by the end of the first year.

At around 18 months, babies begin to feel sensitive to how others perceive them, becoming self-conscious. They are highly sensitive to feelings of shame, especially when adults are harsh with them. Limit setting becomes necessary, but it must be done kindly. The role of the attachment figure is to create an experience of positive regard and attunement for the child.

Nonverbal communications hold sway during this stage, as children at this age are still working mainly from the right brain.

It is not until around 2 years of age that children develop self-awareness and a drive for autonomy. They have a new awareness of their separateness from their caregivers and begin to use words such as "me," "my," and "I." Toddlers are capable of feeling more complex emotions about themselves, such as embarrassment, shame, and pride. When adults accept their children's individuality and directly support their self-directed behavior, they bolster children's budding sense of independence. The role of parents at this phase of development is to sustain a positive attitude toward the children's developing individuation while setting necessary limits with firmness and kindness.

Between 3 and 4 years of age, children start to describe themselves in terms of concrete characteristics. "My name is Jon. I am a boy, and I have a new toy." Positive feedback about their actions and abilities goes a long way to help them develop confidence in their newfound autonomy and eventually in themselves (Brazelton & Sparrow, 2006).

When children are around 5 or 6, they often transition to kindergarten. This transition requires an adjustment to cooperating with others. Children are called upon to think beyond themselves in order to share and be part of a group. Between the ages of 5 and 7 years, children's stories about themselves become richer as memory develops in significant ways. Children can form and recall conscious memories and form ideas about themselves and others.

Temporal memories, which link to specific timelines, appear to form between ages 8 and 11 years, after which stories develop with a better sense of time, place, and person. Across the heart of childhood, the role of parents in facilitating a positive identity is to joyfully mirror children's blossoming abilities and identity, taking care to not overfocus on children's misbehaviors, weaknesses, or failures, and to make limits explicit, reliable, and kindly enforced. With this approach, parents facilitate the development of resilience, which, at its core, is an ability to return to underlying confidence in one's capability and hardiness.

In adolescence, children transition from childhood to adulthood. They shift toward seeking primary support from peers rather than parents, and their still-developing identity becomes increasingly influenced by peer feedback, although the relationship with parents remains influential. Between 12 and 17 years, major changes take place in the brain: neuronal pruning and restructuring for more complex thought (Siegel, 2015; Spear, 2013). Teenagers have a temporary decrease in prefrontal cortex functioning, which controls executive functions such as attention, planning, judgment, impulse control, and decision making. They are also more emotional and driven by limbic reactivity. Their relationships are likely to be more emotionally driven.

While the same parental principles described above for facilitating positive identity remain in place, they can be harder to adhere to with sometimes highly emotional and impulsive teens. A new feature of parenting at this age is the increasing necessity of allowing teens to express their evolving identity in their life choices. The fine line of maintaining safety while respecting a child's self-determination in the shifting and emotionally intense climate of adolescence makes this phase challenging and enlivening.

Older teens and young adults are better able to integrate and master multiple roles than are younger teens as their identity becomes more stable over time. This is the stage of a maturing cerebral and prefrontal cortex. The last portion of the brain to develop is the prefrontal cortex, the seat of higher-level social, moral, and personal functioning. It is the seat of self-control and judgment, which is believed to fully mature by around the age of 30 years (Dubuc, 2013).

In early adulthood, parents still have a consultant role, offering a touchpoint their adult children may turn to for emotional support and guidance. During this phase, parents' deep understanding of their children's history and identity puts them in a unique position to help young adults think about themselves and their decisions. And then, well into our retirement years, we continue to develop wisdom, improved judgment, and empathy.

Creating a healthy identity is a slow and multilayered process that takes decades to complete. It depends on a robust relational start and continues to build across a lifetime. The brain takes about 30 years to fully mature—to become maximally flexible, efficient, and accurate. Parents are necessary participants throughout this long developmental journey, supporting children in building a positive, integrated, and stable sense of self.

5

Problem Scenarios: Unhealthy Attachments and Their Costs

The quality of parent–child attachment is impacted by genetics, parents' experience, and previous generations. Once the child is conceived, the parents and extended family begin to lay a foundation for the attachment process: the groundwork for integrating the new life. Support from friends and family can strengthen new parents in this significant life transition. When parents feel scaffolded by others, they are more able to meet the emotional and physical needs of their newborn. Children's quickly developing brains are directly influenced by these early relationships, primarily at home but also in the community around them.

Parents all come to the job of parenting with their own varied and often checkered attachment histories. Some parents were well parented themselves and luckily dodged or resolved past traumatic experiences; these parents are more likely to embark upon the adventure of parenthood with the necessary tools to intuitively build healthy attachments with their children. Safe, stable, caring parents tend to create secure homes and raise children who grow up to feel secure.

Just over half of the population is believed to fit in the category of secure attachment. As therapists, we rarely meet these parents unless they are raising a child with an innate emotional disturbance or who has experienced trauma. When we do, they are often easy to work with, take guidance well, and can meet their children's needs fairly accurately and consistently. The parents who need our help the most are often struggling to be adequately available and responsive for reasons varying from their own attachment patterns to the real stresses of their lives. More insecure parents tend to create homes that extend feelings of anxiety, tension, avoidance, or chaos to their children; thus, the children are likely to grow up feeling insecure. Add to this the needs of a high-intensity child, and those parents—ideally—reach out to a therapist for help.

The vulnerability of these parents seeking help with their children is worthy of our highest respect. They are making their best effort to heal what is probably the most precious relationship in their lives. Although their interpersonal weaknesses and wounds may be negatively impacting their children, an approach of acceptance and honor instead of blaming and judging will give you the greatest access to the parents' hearts, where real change can occur.

TEMPERAMENT AND ATTACHMENT: MISMATCHES AND STRESS

Individuals are born with different innate temperaments such as boldness, sensitivity, extroversion, and reactivity. Although they do not predict attachment category, variations in temperament can influence attachment development, as can the match or mismatch of temperament between parent and child. The parent and child each bring their own unique qualities to their interactions with each other. Secure attachment between parent and child is built together; it is coconstructed—a two-way interaction.

The parent of a calm child will find it easier to soothe them, and thus can feel positively connected to that child (Tronick, 2017). A parent of an anxious child will find them more difficult to soothe and therefore may feel more stress in the connection. A calm parent will find it is easier to manage their child regardless of the child's temperament, while an anxious or fragile parent will find child-rearing more stressful in and of itself. Adding a challenging child to that family will increase the strain, so more emotional support and parenting skills may be needed for the relationship to thrive. The application of support and parenting skills are detailed in Chapter 6.

Parent–Child Fit

Every child is a genetic roll of the dice. A child may have his mother's hair and his grandfather's height; a child's father's peaceful disposition may be recognizable in her, but something in her sense of humor might be reminiscent of her aunt. Even beyond characteristics that remind us of ourselves or other blood relatives of the child, the possible expressions of a child's genetic makeup are vast. Each ovum has many possible chromosome combinations. So does each sperm. Add to this the not-insignificant effect of the child's environment, and parents can be very surprised as they grow to know their child.

Due to the wealth of possible types, parents will inevitably feel different degrees of rapport, familiarity, and connectedness with each of their children. Parents can easily find themselves raising children that feel very different from them. When there is a match between parent and child, it can lead to wondrous moments of resonance, intuitive understanding, and intimacy. When there is a mismatch, it can be more challenging, but may also offer parents an opportunity to see life differently than they would have otherwise. Dissimilar children can amaze parents with their gifts, provide them with experiences they would never have sought out on their own, and bring new empathy and insight to the parents' worldview.

In the rough and tumble of day-to-day life, however, a mismatch can cause unanticipated stress and struggles to connect. For example, a loud, expressive, and energetic parent of a highly sensitive child may unintentionally overstimulate the child regularly. Such a parent may have difficulty matching her level of stimulation to the receptivity of the child or may have trouble recognizing the child's more subtle expressions of emotions and needs. This parent may need to work hard to match the child's natural pace, to meet her without overwhelming her, and to allow her the time and space she needs to express herself.

Conversely, a highly active, emotionally intense, willful child can be especially challenging for a more sensitive, irritable, or fragile parent, who may be overly stressed by the demands of keeping up with, resonating to, and setting limits with a ball of fire. In these situations, the parent may be tempted to snap at the child, withdraw, or become overly accommodating or permissive to avoid the stress of conflict, when what the child may actually need is to have his intensity appreciated, matched, and guided.

Connecting with a child healthily and harmoniously is easy in theory and harder in practice. It can be quite tricky when a parent must leave her comfort zone to resonate with a child and to match their energy and sensibilities. However, in these moments of disconnection or tension, it's so important to see the child accurately, respect the child's natural pace and rhythm, and move with them, not against them.

Slowing and quieting when a sensitive child needs more space or time or allowing for exuberance or rage in an intense child can be difficult for parents whose constitutions or histories bring up resistance. Ultimately, however, it's worth the work, as it communicates to the child that their natural style of being is just fine. When a parent is able, more often than not, to pull off this feat, they have given the child two of the most important gifts parents can give to children: the gift of feeling lovable, and of knowing that others can be trusted.

FAMILY CHANGES: SEPARATION AND LOSS

Children are highly reliant on those close to them to feel contained, seen, and emotionally held. When family constellations and familiar patterns of relationships change, children's attachment systems are strained. They are likely to feel less secure.

Even very young children feel a sense of loss when separated from someone in their family. Children of all ages react with grief and feelings of insecurity when a member of their clan dies. While parents sometimes think the loss of a grandparent will not impact little children, this is not usually so. Even if the grandparent is only an acquaintance, children perceive and react to the parents' grief, making that loss resonate throughout the family system. In the wake of a death, children may sense decreased emotional availability from family members, and may have to struggle with the typical questions provoked by the awareness of death. This struggle may manifest as clinginess, neediness, and anxiety as they wrestle with these questions and with the complexity of their own grief and the grief of others they love.

In cases of divorce, children only rarely lose a parent. Still, divorce means a dramatic change in the day-to-day fabric of children's lives, and this can provoke feelings of sadness, fear, instability, and confusion. Questions arise for children during separation and divorce: questions around security, around whether they are to blame, around whether a parent will cease to love them or be there for them in the way they need. At these times, parents are often preoccupied with their own feelings and with the stress of adjusting to single parenting. It is common for parents to be less emotionally available to children and less emotionally stable during the adjustment.

Perhaps surprisingly, the addition of a new family member can also be stressful to children. Although most people consider a remarriage or the birth or adoption of a new sibling to be a cause for celebration, these events also have a ripple effect that can impact children positively and negatively. When attention is necessarily diverted to the new family member, vulnerable children may respond with any of a number of negative emotions, including insecure thoughts and feelings—for example, feeling unimportant, displaced, or needy.

NEGATIVE INFLUENCE ON CHILDREN'S IDENTITIES

Just as the attachment relationship is a crucible for building positive identity and self-esteem in a child, it can also be the source of a negative sense of self. Children develop a sense of who they are in the context of their early relationships. The verbal and nonverbal communication children receive from significant others informs them that they are seen as good or bad, fun or dull, bright or slow. This feedback can outweigh children's direct observations and experiences of success or failure. Each bit of information they receive in their interactions with significant adults is filed away as kernels of truth about who they are. Over time, these data points are consolidated and used to form children's growing identities (Baylin & Hughes, 2016; Brazelton & Greenspan, 2001; Medina, 2014; Siegel, 2020; Winnicott, 1964/1992).

Interestingly, one's sense of identity is not always accurate. With consistent erroneous feedback, children can build faulty beliefs about themselves: for example, that they are selfish when, in truth, they are generous, or that they are weak when they are actually strong. This pattern underscores the fact that identity is a result of feedback from the world as much as it is a result of accurate self-assessment.

Self-Defeating Stories

Unfortunately, parents often try to shape children's behavior by pointing out to them when they are off track, and this can shape identity in ways that are unintended. Conventional parenting models teach generosity by scolding children when they don't share, encourage honesty by confronting children when they are lying, or attempt to foster responsibility with statements such as, "You are so irresponsible!" The problem with this intervention is that it inadvertently promotes a negative sense of self.

A child who consistently hears that they are rude does not necessarily learn to be polite. Instead, they learn that they are rude. These corrections tend to occur when the child has just failed to be polite, so the comment sinks in that much deeper because it is backed up by incontrovertible fact. The child takes it in as an experience of failure, and the experience goes into their stock of self-information as a data point: "I am not very polite. Politeness is not one of my assets." This self-perception of rudeness can become a self-fulfilling prophecy.

As we know, self-image is a self-perpetuating set of beliefs. Just as individuals who believe they are funny are comfortable telling a joke, and are likely to do so often, individuals who think they're boring will feel uncomfortable taking the floor and try to avoid it. Parents can inadvertently build negative identities when they, for example, repeatedly criticize their children for being disorganized and point out their disorganization. Even with the good intention of teaching organization, they insert into children's identities, "I am a disorganized person. I'm just not good at getting organized." When verbally abused children repeatedly hear that they are stupid, they are likely to believe it—to interpret their life as the life of a stupid person and assume that their choices are probably wrong.

Of course, children with experiences of failure and a resulting negative story will tend to avoid situations where they do not feel successful. This avoidance, unfortunately, creates a problematic cycle. What these children are avoiding out of fear of failure is precisely the thing that they need to address, but they cannot work on it naturally due to being stuck in a cycle of fear, avoidance, and failure. A key to changing this negative cycle is breaking the pattern through experiences of success and recognition.

MISTREATMENT: ABUSE AND NEGLECT

Just as speaking critically to a child can have unintended negative consequences for the child, other patterns of negativity can also have long-lasting ill effects. While relational conflict is unavoidable, extreme conflict can lead to harm. Most parents do not intentionally create harmful environments for children, but when parents find themselves under extreme levels of stress or burdened by their own emotional issues, abusive behaviors can result.

The mistreatment of children through emotional or physical abuse requires immediate intervention. Exposure to abuse can have long-term emotional and physical consequences, including disorganized attachment. Angry, hostile adults at home create an environment of fear and insecurity. When children are mistreated or hurt by their caregivers, they learn that their potential sources of comfort and security are also sources of pain. This confusing experience leads to a pattern of contradictory and distrustful feelings toward adults—not just toward the abusive parents. Mistreated children will automatically interact with others in the ways they learned in the context of the abusive relationship. Even if the abuse was early in childhood and children have no conscious memory of it, they implicitly feel that people are not reliably safe.

Neglect is a form of child maltreatment and can take many forms. Obviously, parents or guardians who fail to provide food, safe housing, education, or medical care to children in their care are considered neglectful. Other, more subtle forms of neglect include lack of supervision or emotional presence. In homes where parents are not physically and emotionally available, warm, or stable, children feel insecure and anxious (Main & Hesse, 1990; Parkes et al., 2006; Schore, 2001). This does not imply that parents must be attuned 24/7, but it does mean that day to day, children need a consistent and caring adult presence (Brazelton & Greenspan, 2001; Winnicott, 1964/1992).

Neglectful homes leave children feeling vulnerable, alone, fearful, and unworthy of love. When children have experienced neglect, they may learn their attachment cues are useless, and come to believe that comfort is not available to them. Also, they may learn that support is not provided to serve their needs; rather, it is provided unpredictably. The child may internalize this as a sense of being unworthy of care or as a sense of adults being unreliable and uncaring. Their essential attachment needs are not being met.

In some cases, parents instinctively avoid emotional connections with their children because children's primitive emotional and physical needs trigger the parents' feelings of vulnerability. This adverse reaction to children's immature and dependent emotions may be due to the parents' own painful histories of neglect or abuse. This type of parental avoidance can be improved through individual therapeutic work with the parents. By providing a secure therapeutic relationship to the parent, a therapist can effectively improve parents' ability to connect emotionally with their child—which, in turn, can increase parents' stability, promote feelings of hope, reduce overall stress, and increase the sense of safety in the home (Davidson & McEwen, 2012; Levine, 2015; Saunders et al., 2011; Siegel & Hartzell, 2013; Wallin, 2007).

We know that secure parenting has a powerful positive effect on brain development, and that chronic adversity can interfere with healthy brain growth. A stressful home environment can cause brain structures to adapt in ways that may help children survive in the current situation but may cause problems in the future. Children's brains are shaped by their experiences in ways that can help or hinder them throughout their lives (McGreevy, 2011; Schore, 2015; Siegel, 2020; Singleton et al., 2014). Parents can, at any time, make positive changes to improve their availability for attachment and build a healthier home environment. Trauma, abuse, and recovery or adaptations to adversity are discussed in more detail in Part III.

MISLEADING BEHAVIORS AND ATTACHMENT ISSUES

When the attachment relationship has gone awry, therapists may see children whose behaviors are erratic, chaotic, or irrational. These children may be aggressive or withdrawn; they may not read nonverbal cues well or may seem to fail to perceive the feelings and reactions of others. These children may also have difficulty regulating their emotions and bodies. As a result, they may overreact or underreact to pain, hunger, and emotion. They often seem impulsive. These behavioral patterns can interfere with the development of positive connections with others. At the core of these widely varying difficulties is a weakness in the children's *internal working model* of themselves and their attachment figures.

This internal working model is a set of expectations people have about who they are, what others are like, and how interactions are likely to unfold. This internalized model organizes self-awareness and expectations of others. In children with attachment issues, this model does not function smoothly—and can guide their behavior toward self-defeating patterns that do not reliably produce loving reactions from those around them.

Such children can be confusing to their parents, as they often miscue them. They don't give the same clear-cut attachment signals that well-nurtured children can provide. For example, when parents approach or offer connection, the child may turn away, express disinterest or boredom, or respond with hostility. On the other hand, they may demand contact and seem to crave attention greedily, but do not feel genuinely connected when parents respond. As a result, parents may have difficulty feeling bonded to and favorable toward that child.

Keep in mind the point made earlier: The attachment relationship is coconstructed. It is a product of both children's and parents' attachment expectations, behaviors, and emotions. Creating attachment is easier for parents when they feel some connection. The parents' sense of connection is enhanced by eye contact with children, the children initiating physical contact, their positive facial expressions, and their responsiveness to suggestions from the parents. When these are absent or fail to meet with parental expectations or desires, parents have a harder time feeling connected. Even parents with a healthily functioning attachment system may have strong reactions to these children. They may feel unable to attach to them or feel confused or irritated by them. It is common to feel rejected, hurt, frightened, or overwhelmed by these children.

Still, regardless of a child's history, resilient and loving parents can make all the difference. When parents take on a therapeutic parenting role, change can occur. Parents hold the potential to change the life trajectories of children with painful early experiences. New and healthier attachments can be formed over time.

NEED FOR INTERVENTION AND GOOD NEWS ABOUT RECOVERY

Early intervention is critical if the parent–child relationships are unsafe or neglectful. Sometimes it is necessary to move children to safer environments, at least temporarily, for them to heal and return to a healthier developmental path. Repair is possible at any age, but the quicker the intervention for safety, the better. Beginning this process early in life takes advantage of the greatest flexibility in terms of neurological, physiological, and emotional development (Cramer et al., 2011).

Investigations into the effect of chaotic, crowded, or conflict-heavy environments on children's stress hormones show a significant impact on children's biological indicators of stress—particularly when a child's parents are inattentive or unresponsive (Blair, 2008). These elevated levels of stress hormones (in particular, cortisol) harm the developing brain. The good news, however, is that when parents are sensitive and attentive even in times of adversity, their children show almost no biological indicators of stress. To quote Paul Tough (2012), "High-quality mothering [parenting], in other words, can act as a powerful buffer against the damage that adversity inflicts on a child's stress-response system."

Parental attunement and availability can buffer and repair the effects of environmental stress. What a powerful statement! The research is clear: Early experiences of nurturance create the biological milieu that makes resilience possible in stressful situations.

6

Treatment Interventions: Repairing Attachments and Building Security

Now that we have reviewed what can go right or wrong in early attachment, we will discuss the stance and perspective we recommend providers take when working with families with general emotional or behavioral problems, or with attachment disruptions at the level of the parents or the children.

Here, we discuss the emotional context of doing attachment work with families, including raising awareness of family vulnerabilities and potential pitfalls. This context sets providers up to conceptualize their intervention with a family and begin to help them move in a secure direction. Specific tools for this work are offered later in this chapter.

REAL-LIFE PARENTING, STRESS, AND SELF-CARE

Primary in the care of struggling families is encouraging parents to care for themselves. When adults add children to their lives, their lives change completely. They gain some things (an expanded sense of family, new depths of emotion) and lose others (access to private time, time with their partner, and the ease of prioritizing their own wants and needs) (Kabat-Zinn, 2005; Medina, 2014). Adjustment to this new state can be a jolt. Often, people focus so intently on celebrating a new child and adjusting to caring for them that the losses are not acknowledged or mourned. In light of all this change, it is no wonder parents often wake up years later unsure how they became so stressed, isolated, and physically depleted. When parents add children with a history of adversity to their family, the adjustment to parenting can be even more intense, challenging, and at times overwhelming. For many parents, taking the time and energy to nourish and recharge themselves can seem like time and energy they can ill afford to spend.

For therapists working with children, taking into account parents' levels of stress and emotional states and their ability to care for themselves is an essential starting point, particularly as we work to avoid the pitfall of treating the child in isolation. In addition to the strain of caring for struggling or difficult children, parents who neglect themselves—failing to get adequate sleep, exercise, social connection, and fun because they prioritize their parental responsibilities far above their self-care—pay the price themselves, and that cost ultimately trickles down to their children.

Helping parents to focus on their own needs increases their resources for helping their children and their ability to work with the therapist toward the end of improving family life and well-being. Prioritizing one's self can be difficult during times of intense family pressure, but parents can get in front of it by committing to even a few minutes a day for themselves. Grounded and well-cared-for parents will find it easier to bring connection, thoughtfulness, and warmth to their families.

GOOD ENOUGH PARENTS

Many years ago, Daniel Winnicott, a renowned British psychoanalyst, developed the idea of the "good enough parent." This concept acknowledges that all parents are flawed and addresses the fear that parents may ruin their children with imperfect approaches to parenting. According to Winnicott (1953, 1964/1992), children only require their caretaking to be "good enough," which is usually sensitive, usually responsive, and usually accurate to the children's needs. The occasional error can be taken in stride by the healthy child and will not necessarily damage them.

Many cultures encourage the impossible fantasy of the perfect and selfless parent. Straining for perfection is not only stressful to real-life parents—it is also hard on their children. Helping parents develop defenses against unhelpful and negative social pressures, criticism, and self-recrimination can lessen these unhealthy strivings.

When children experience their parents overworking, grasping, and tense, they pick up that stress. Parents parenting from this place model dissatisfaction and failure to accept their natural limitations and imperfections—the inability to accept reality.

It does the child no good to be the only imperfect person in the relationship. Perfect parents do not exist, and children do not need their parents to be perfect. Nevertheless, children do best when parents interact warmly, attempt to comfort their children when upset, show interest in their children, attune to the children's needs and emotional states, and discipline calmly.

BEGINNING TO MEND ATTACHMENTS: PARENTS AND CHILDREN

Attachment patterns can be influenced or even mended in childhood and also in adulthood. Parents who have insecure attachment patterns can develop a stronger sense of security through positive, attuned relationships later in life (Saunders et al., 2011). As a result of time spent in a healthy relationship, their attachment strategy can shift from insecure to a more secure strategy called *earned secure*. Earned security can develop in adulthood in the context of a loving friendship or marriage. Successful psychotherapy can also impact the attachment system positively and foster improved relational security. Through psychotherapy, or a process of deep self-reflection, a person can create a better understanding of their past attachment experiences and shift into a more secure attachment strategy.

Studies have found that parents with earned security are more likely to raise secure children than are parents with unresolved insecure histories (Saunders et al., 2011; Siegel & Hartzell, 2013). Although attaining earned security can lead to more positive relationships, it does not erase old feelings of hurt or loss. Some of the old insecurity may still exist; however, it can be lessened and the person can go forward to develop satisfying adult connections and raise securely attached children.

When parents are raising children who have had early attachment disruptions, they have an entirely different experience than when raising healthy newborn children, or adopted children with a strong attachment start. The good news is that therapists can remind parents that they are in the best position to stabilize and mend children's attachment relationship systems; and that there is always the potential for change, even with more intractable attachment patterns.

Remember, the attachment relationship is created by more than the parents; it is coconstructed. The parent–child attachment is a product of both the parent's and the child's past attachment experiences, expectations, and behaviors. Parents can learn to interact in ways that are likely to engage children's attention and interest. Parents may need help learning to reach out to their children, where they are, to foster relatedness in the current moment.

Parents can begin by trying these practices:

- Use the child's name warmly.
- Use "we" and "us" frequently.
- Refer to common history.
- Remain available, neither escalating nor withdrawing when problems arise.
- Maintain positive nonverbal expressions.
- Communicate to the child what the parent understands about them.
- Allow the child to correct parents if they disagree with parents' understanding of them.
- Express interest verbally and nonverbally: Look at the child, focus on their behavior and speech, remain present in a relaxed and calm manner.
- Pace the child: Avoid rushing the child.
- Mirror the child's movements and sounds (but not when the child is dysregulated).

There is a delicate balance in making one's attachment presence felt without intruding. The task of parents is to make continued efforts to connect, learn what type of experiences are more welcomed by the child, and attend to their cues to back off. Therapists can help parents understand that their child may miscue them—for example, that they may push the parent away when they actually want the parent to stay, or draw the parent in when they really need more space. Parents can only understand this miscuing by trial and error, so they need to be patient with themselves and their children in the learning process. It is the parent's job to stay attuned to the child's emotions and help them learn to identify feelings and express their needs more directly over time.

Remember, healthy attachment patterns are fostered by parental positivity and consistency. Children with problematic attachment histories have had erratic caregiving or negative experiences in the hands of caregivers. Alteration of the child's assumptions about intimate caregiving relationships can occur when parents are uniformly kind, regularly attuned, and mostly predictable. Consistency in parenting can be seen as parents acting and reacting in the same way as much as possible. Through consistency, the child learns what to expect from their parents. If adults' reactions are the same each time, the child will not have to worry about what they will do and can begin to trust.

THERAPEUTIC ATTACHMENT: ATTUNEMENT AND CLEAR BOUNDARIES

The therapeutic guidance above creates an inviting relational pattern with the potential for healing. An attuned, empathic connection develops from the parents' abilities to read, understand, and resonate with their children. To attach in a healthy way and heal from past negative experiences, the child needs to feel resonance at a verbal and nonverbal level.

An attuned parent–child connection does not mean that children can have whatever they want whenever they want it, but rather that when adults set a limit, they can accept and acknowledge children's feelings in response to the situation. Some children with complicated histories have learned that manipulation is the most effective way to get what they want and need. Allowing this pattern to continue through overindulgence or unwillingness to set limits is gratifying to children at the moment—but it reinforces manipulation and does not change unhealthy habits.

A primary goal of therapeutic parenting is to hold limits consistently and predictably while allowing children to be disappointed in the moment and being willing to be present to that disappointment in a caring way (the heart of parenting). This is what will lead to a more authentic connection.

ATTACHMENT-SOUND PARENTING AND THE NURTURED HEART APPROACH

Howard Glasser's books *Transforming the Difficult Child: The Nurtured Heart Approach* and *The Transforming the Intense Child Workbook* offer sound therapeutic interventions to help parents build secure attachments (Glasser & Easley, 2016; Glasser & Lowenstein, 2017; Hektner et al., 2013). We recommend that therapists teach parents this approach early in treatment for implementation at home. In many cases, this leads to a profound shift in the parent–child relationship and the emotional tone of the household, which in turn impacts the children's emotional states and behaviors. This simple step can sometimes be all that is needed to achieve the family's treatment goals, with no further treatment required.

This model recommends an interactive style that is a powerful example of attachment-sound parenting and that builds on the creation of trust in the parent–child relationship and the development of positive identity for the child. These aims are accomplished as parents follow these guidelines: (1) reliably not overreacting to children's errors and misbehaviors, (2) reliably responding with interest and warmth to children, and (3) reliably being clear and consistent regarding what is expected of children. These three concepts, which are consistent with attachment-sound parenting, are referred to as *The 3 Stands*.

The 3 Stands of the Nurtured Heart Approach

These guidelines are the foundation of NHA's style of relationship-based parenting. They are commitments parents and caregivers are encouraged to make for the well-being of their children and family. Taking a stand means being committed to a position and holding it firmly even in the face of adversity. It is a means of being steady and grounded in a perspective one feels is right, and not wavering. We will revisit the 3 Stands throughout this book; for this discussion of attachment repair and the building of security, we focus primarily on Stands 1 and 2 (Glasser & Easley, 2016; Glasser & Lowenstein, 2017).

Stand 1: *Absolutely No.* Absolutely No means taking a stand that absolutely no reactive energy is available to the child for negativity. Adults strive to respond to misbehavior with neutrality. This stand encompasses several concepts, including:

- Maintaining parental calm in the face of problems
- Not overreacting to misconduct; rather, reacting mildly—particularly in the heat of the moment
- Not tuning in with particular interest or curiosity to children's failures
- Bringing down one's level of energy and focus when negativity is present

Consistent use of Stand 1 is an effective way to increase safety and trust within the parent–child relationship. It creates an environment in which children learn they can count on their parents to be calm and regulated. By employing this Stand, parents can avoid mutual escalations common in families. It serves to model respect and emotional regulation.

A second advantage of Stand 1 is its effectiveness at focusing children on their innate goodness—by avoiding reinforcement of negative messages they may have internalized about themselves. When parents can respond mildly to problems, they effectively undercut the negative feedback children often receive about their failures. Where negative feedback inadvertently strengthens the child's negative view of themselves, a more neutral response effectively stops fueling negative identity.

Child therapists are trained to reflect what children are feeling and doing as a means of expressing attunement and compassion. This process helps to show children that they are seen and understood, which is an empathic approach. However, therapists can often reflect somewhat indiscriminately. To positively impact children's identities, our reflections need to be accurately focused on children's excellence of character or positive choices.

Remember your early play therapy training: Never reflect behaviors that you don't want to see again.

Stand 2: Absolutely Yes. Absolutely Yes means an absolutely enthusiastic and consistently positive response to the child for any form of success. It expresses a determined effort on the part of parents to sincerely highlight and celebrate anything children do that is not problematic. This stand is implemented by:

- Verbally and physically interacting warmly and enthusiastically with children whenever they are on track
- Lowering the bar on the definition of success so that children experience feedback for success more often
- Creating a rich "time-in" of fun, connection, and praise that forms a steady backdrop in children's lives

Therapists can recommend parents implement this stand by frequently giving their children positive verbal recognitions. Both the substance (positive acknowledgment for even minor successes) and the timing (often, and in moments when no rules are being broken) of these recognitions demonstrate to the children that they are worthy of adult attention, valued by their parents, and on track.

These recognitions take the form of clearly articulating to the child what the parent sees them feeling and doing, for example, "I see you watching a cartoon; you are lying calmly on the couch and giggling and giggling." Or, "You seem angry now; you are telling me how you feel and using your words." This type of affirmation requires attentive connection—being with the child in the moment. It expresses attunement through specific, detailed descriptions of the child's current state. What has passed is no longer relevant; what may happen in the future is not the point. The successful Stand 2 recognition is about what is going well right now.

To be effective, parental recognitions can be given one to several times an hour and are best taken in by children when they are detailed and given with a bit of enthusiasm. They should always focus on what is good at this moment. Recognitions should incorporate congruent body language and tone of voice; when giving a recognition, it is critical to show caring and pleasure with facial expression, eye contact, tone of voice, gesture, and posture. Incongruent body language will hit children's radar and weaken feelings of trust. For children who are on the go and don't stick around long enough for a detailed recognition, a mere "wonderful cooperation" may be all the parents can get in, so they need to be sure to pair it with highly positive physical expressions of delight.

Recognitions increase children's trust in their parents and increase their belief that they are on-track, worthy, and valued. Any time is a good time for recognition—even, or perhaps especially, when children are upset. Angry feelings need to be seen and accepted too. At these times, paying attention to what children are doing right and how they are feeling can calm them and foster attachment and pride. One caution, however, is never to use recognitions with behavior the parents hope not to see again, as it will reinforce those behaviors. Specific use of recognitions for teaching and discipline are described in detail in Part IV.

If parents can find anything positive in the moment—which, with practice, will be almost always—then, by all means, they should say it. For attachment building, the sincerity of recognitions is essential. When parents can dig deep and get in touch with their genuine appreciation for what they see in their children, the resulting recognitions are imbued with power, attunement, and authenticity that fosters secure emotions in children. Being in a receptive state helps parents to do this with accuracy and sincerity. This feeling of being seen and valued is at the core of attachment security.

Stand 3: *Absolutely Clear.* Absolutely Clear advises parents to be absolutely predictable in response to the child. This third Stand works cooperatively with the first two to create stability and predictability in the parent–child relationship, even when times are difficult.

This stand is implemented by:

- Defining rules and expectations in a way that is completely clear to parents and children
- Reliably responding to children with connection and interest and positive verbal and physical interactions when children are within bounds
- Invariably responding to misbehavior, regardless of the size, with calm limit setting

Absolutely Clear is a way of removing the gray areas from children's lives. Improved clarity not only increases children's understanding of the rules, but increases their willingness to live from the powerful position of cooperation and being true to their positive selves. When applied faithfully, Absolutely Clear also decreases counterproductive adult behavior that can unintentionally reinforce misconduct.

Once Stands 1 and 2 are in place, the establishment of clarity and limit setting is possible. Stand 3 is described in more detail in Part IV of this book (Table 6.1).

Table 6.1 THE NURTURED HEART APPROACH: THE 3 STANDS		
Stand 1 Absolutely No	Stand 2 Absolutely Yes	Stand 3 Absolutely Clear
No energy for problems: Adults remain calm and neutral in the face of problems. They do not focus on negativity, errors, or misbehavior with any energy.	Yes to any success: Adults intentionally focus on and respond enthusiastically to any success, no matter how small. They demonstrate interest and authentic recognition to any moment the child is on track.	Clarity at all times: Adults communicate and calmly hold clear boundaries. Limit setting is low in intensity and lacks any inadvertent relational reward.
Reliably not overreacting to children's errors and misbehaviors.	Reliably responding to children with interest and enthusiasm.	Reliably being clear and consistent regarding what is expected of children.

SOURCE: © Howard Glasser, Creator/Developer of the Nurtured Heart Approach

BUILDING A POSITIVE STORY

As mentioned earlier, children build their identities from their experiences, self-observation, and the feedback they get from others. This knowledge gives family therapists an opening that can be used to influence self-image positively. As parents are in a prime position to help with this work, we recommend that therapists begin treatment of children by guiding parents to promote positive identity by not overreacting to children's errors and insistently, enthusiastically pointing out both small and large successes. The child's identity as good is dependent on their caretakers' acceptance and validation of their strengths.

Our stories and beliefs about ourselves are stored in our memory, and they are not static like a photo or document: They are changeable. Research shows that a specific memory is revised every time we recall it. Once an event is recalled, the original memory is replaced with a newly revised version of the memory. What we call recall is the most recent version of a memory, not the original (Lee et al., 2017).

Our stories about ourselves can change also. If the feedback from our experiences and the reactions of others are inconsistent with our existing sense of self, our identity can shift. With regular and consistent feedback, our identity will change to integrate the new information. This window of change is our opening for positive growth.

Parents in a negative state can become stuck in complaint and judgment. Negative messages can cycle in their minds and interfere with the awareness needed to take a balanced stance. Helping parents drop out of this anxious cycle and into their bodily emotions is usually best accomplished through guiding them to become more self-aware (recognizing that they are in a negative state) and to then consciously move away from negative thoughts. This mental shift brings parents into a reflective, mindful state. Once parents are more present in the session, they can accept positive recognition of their own successes: making efforts to break a negative pattern, coming to appointments, or doing better than they did last month. Then, parents are ready to look at the positive and create recognitions for their children.

Once parents can see their children's successes, we want them to tune in to their appreciation of those successes and acknowledge them out loud with their children, even in difficult times. Encourage them to include acknowledgment of the intrinsic qualities the child is displaying while engaging in the desired behavior. The framework can look something like this:

1. Statement of the behavior being observed: "I see you sharing your cars with your brother."

2. Reference to the intrinsic positive quality reflected in the behavior: "That shows your kindness and generosity."

This skill is probably familiar to therapists because it is commonly used to reflect clients' feelings or successes back to them. Parents are less likely to be immediately adept with this type of reflective speech and may need specific guidance, homework to practice, and recognition of their own growing success.

Devote Therapy Time to Reviewing and Celebrating Successes

We recommend using the therapy appointment as a time to review and celebrate children's successes. Spend the bulk of time in therapy with parents and children modeling and coaching nurturing interactions rather than dissecting the errors or problems of the week. This can feel like a tall order to the therapist at first, as focus on problems and problem solving is a major part of the standard model most therapists learn in their training; but our experience suggests that focusing on problems does not build children's confidence—nor does it strengthen the connection and attunement between parents and children that fosters the building of secure attachment.

In individual child therapy, we want to use both Stands 1 and 2 (absolutely no energy to negativity and high energy to success). Therapists can encourage this in parents in session by pointing out children's assets and positive behaviors so that they can be taken in as successes. Begin sessions with a question like, "What went well for you this week?" or "Tell me about a success you have had recently." Take initiative to articulate successes you hear children alluding to. Children do not always take in the major victory that it is to avoid an argument, to make it to school when not in the mood, or to complete a chore in spite of not wanting to. A therapist who remains alert to these overlooked successes can contribute to children's growing sense of positive self-image by overtly and warmly highlighting this point of view in session. Discussion of virtues and values, and of times the children have manifested these in the waiting room or in session, can also be powerful.

> **AVOID THE TOXIC POSITIVITY OR POLLYANNA APPROACH**
>
> While we highly recommend Stand 2, Absolutely Yes, in parenting and psychotherapy, the Pollyanna approach—abundant, overblown recognitions that are dismissive of feelings, without depth, or given inauthentically—do not work. Model giving recognitions grounded in the absolute truth of the moment. Recognize successes from an authentic, heart-centered space, and be sensitive to proper timing of those recognitions.

Building Positive Identity With Stands 1 and 2: A Closer Look

In individual psychotherapy, NHA has an impact at behavioral, cognitive, and relational levels. Behaviorally, warm recognition can serve as encouragement to repeat the behavior responded to. Cognitively, it can help children develop new thinking patterns about themselves: "Like he said, I *did* hold the door open. I guess I am a kind person." Relationally, it can create an experience of a safe and attuned relationship in which children feel valued, appreciated, and seen in a positive light.

Have parents start by implementing Stand 1 with no reactive energy to negativity. For this stand to be effective, parents must be able to manage their own emotions and behavior while their children are acting out, misbehaving, or challenging them. For some parents, merely pointing out that yelling and lecturing are ineffective is enough to actualize them to take an immediate step that creates improvement. For other parents, particularly those with their own attachment or emotion management challenges, it will take time to build up the ability to not react with intense energy, passion, and attention to problem behaviors.

To support positive identity in children, it is also necessary to implement Stand 2 energy and enthusiasm for successes. For some parents who are entrenched in negativity, disappointment, or hurt, simply generating awareness of children's successes is a significant piece of emotional work. How do therapists help parents to see their children in a positive light? It often requires the parents to receive some attunement and support—perhaps in their own therapy, if not in the context of the family consultation.

Encourage families to share this new way of interacting with the child with other caregivers, including teachers and extended family. Imagine the power generated when many important adults in children's lives hold them in high regard, reflect their assets and successes back to them, and stringently refuse to identify them by their errors or failings!

Adjusting a Child's Narrative: Building Positive Identity With the Nurtured Heart Approach

Who children think they are will strongly influence what they choose to do and how they choose to act. Whether through criticism or acknowledgment of success, our experiences become stories, which then become our identity. The good news is that our identities can be shifted and changed; they are very responsive to the daily input we receive, especially for children. Regular, accurate, and positive feedback is healing. Ultimately, children will live up to their own view of who they are, positive or negative.

As an attachment intervention, NHA directly addresses the building blocks of a child's identity. Adults foster children's positive identity by pointing out incontrovertible reasons for them to feel good about themselves. Howard Glasser refers to this as "recognizing greatness." For some children—those who are obviously good kids—this is easy. For others, it requires dedication and persistence.

Consider children who have regular angry outbursts, yell, complain, and even hit others. These children have gotten repeated feedback that they are out of control, not likable, and have a terrible temper. Teaching children self-control by criticizing their loss of control does not work; it merely perpetuates their view of themselves as bad kids with lousy self-control. On the other hand, if adults wait to praise them until they handle frustration perfectly, they might be waiting until they are 30. A more effective strategy is for parents to watch for tiny, tiny instances of self-control and comment on those. For example, "You love chocolate chip cookies, and there is a whole plate of them here. You just took two and left some for me. That shows consideration and excellent self-control."

Parents may need to consider lowering the bar on their definition of self-control so that children have a fighting chance of getting over it. If they want to build children's positive identity or create a positive identity for children who believe they are bad, an effective way is for parents to relentlessly search for moments of success, however small, and to appreciate them and bring them to their children's attention, all while refusing to overreact to children's failings. This process is an example of Stand 2, Absolutely Yes. Adults are building a positive identity by giving children frequent positive verbal recognitions, which reveal their truly wonderful characteristics, underline them, celebrate them, and make clear that these qualities truly represent them.

Creating a Coherent Narrative for Healing

Keep in mind that children's stories or narratives about their lives are the threads that help them to make sense of their lives over time. These stories link their life experiences together and are at the root of their identity. When children's stories about themselves and their lives are organized, consistent, and clear, the stories are described as coherent. Sometimes, however, children's stories are spotty or not well integrated. This makes it hard for children to feel a stable self-awareness of who they are and where they came from, and to imagine their future.

Parents can help their children build a clear and cohesive story of who they are and what their lives have been so far. These narratives are easily created if their early lives were safe and secure and their parents have discussed life events, shared memories, and family photos. In this context, positive and coherent stories will develop naturally. Reminiscence is a way to keep children's histories alive in their minds. Different family members will remember and emphasize different aspects of their lives. Children will form their own version of their history over time.

In children with disruptions in early life, such as traumas or adoption, this sense of coherence and flow is diminished. If their lives have been chaotic or traumatic, their life narratives are inconsistent and disorganized or have missing parts. These children's histories can include faulty attributions, some of which fuel negative views of themselves or the world. Reworking and reorganizing these stories can be healing when it corrects self-blame and integrates traumatic memories and emotions.

For many teens and adults, faulty narratives can be corrected by talking it out—over and over again, if necessary—in a safe and supportive environment. The details of the incorrect story can be recognized, explored, and reconsidered. While people's perspectives should be respected, they can also be called into question—particularly when they hold unfair or negative messages about the self. Therapy offers a place for these supportive dialogues to happen, a chance to review and integrate life experiences without judgment, to reorder those stories, and to respond to them emotionally and logically.

In children, new narratives can be created through discussing their memories, sharing common memories, clarifying life stories, organizing and filling in gaps, adding positives where they are lacking, and correcting misconceptions. Art and sand tray work can be helpful therapy supplements. However, for younger children, talking is less effective. Adding play, projective games, photographs, art, and the creation of life books can create clear and coherent stories out of chaotic or spotty histories.

It is important to note that in cases of more severe trauma, the building of a trauma narrative should be delayed until children have learned and are able to use self-soothing and regulating skills. First, teach skills such as deep breathing and progressive muscle relaxation. Next keep in mind that, regardless of age, top-down processing with language and conversation may fail to access the injury in a healing way (Levine, 2015; Ogden & Fisher, 2015; van der Kolk, 2015). In these cases, children can respond positively to physical treatments that utilize bottom-up processing (mindfulness training for children; sensory–motor integration therapy, trauma-informed yoga, Theraplay®, or biofeedback).

MINDFUL PARENTING AND ATTACHMENT

> Indeed I would define mental health as the capacity to be aware of
> the gap between stimulus and response, together with the capacity
> to use this gap constructively.
>
> ROLLO MAY, *FREEDOM AND RESPONSIBILITY RE-EXAMINED*

Raising children, like everything else, is done best with conscious attention
and thoughtfulness. When any relationship is engaged in this thoughtful
way, it increases the capacity to attune, soothe, and educate. Any construc-
tive parenting approach will ask caregivers to be aware of their thoughts
and actions with their children. This mindful intention is at the heart of all
healthy attachments: paying attention to what is essential in the relationship, doing what one believes is right, and aligning with one's values rather
than just reacting.

Mindful parents are, by definition, emotionally present, receptive, and
patient as they support and teach their children (Burke, 2010; Coatsworth
et al., 2009; Duncan et al., 2009; van de Weijer-Bergsma et al., 2012). A
mindful style requires parents to pay attention, on purpose, nonjudgmentally, in the moment. Being intentional in their raising of children allows the
formation of a secure attachment (Cozolino, 2014; Goodman, 2016; Siegel,
2017; Siegel & Hartzell, 2013). Clinicians can guide parents to develop a
mindful approach to their caregiver role. The Nurtured Heart Approach is,
at its center, a mindful approach to parenting.

Teachings on mindfulness have been around since the beginning of
recorded history and are part of our inheritance of philosophy, ethics, and
spirituality. Within these disciplines, priority is placed on self-awareness
and thoughtful interaction with others. Adults who have learned such basic
principles of how to treat others embody them in their lives and pass them
on to children.

Therapists can also apply mindful reflection in their work. A thoughtful
and reflective approach allows us to be cognitively and emotionally present,
creating a sense of security with families. In a mindful therapeutic relationship, therapists keep in mind their clients' thoughts and feelings while also

attending to their own. This stance can help move clients out of negative thought cycles and into a bodily sense of calm and presence and provides great role modeling for parents.

A mindfulness program for parents, studied by Coatsworth et al. (2009), includes these five skills: (1) listening with full attention; (2) nonjudgmental acceptance of self and child; (3) emotional awareness of self and child; (4) self-regulation in the parenting relationship; and (5) compassion for self and child. These skills were found to increase the parents' thoughtful and patient interactions with their children, enhance the parent–child connection, and increase effective parenting strategies. Parents using this approach also reported increased positive child behaviors at home.

Parents can bring mindful attention to their families through emotional sensitivity and acceptance. Accepting parenting does not mean that anything goes—rather, it means that parents are aware of children's errors and set limits without being critical or defensive. Acceptance means parents may reject a specific behavior but never insult the child. Mindful parenting is nonjudgmental in terms of love and respect for children, but it does allow for seeing problems that arise and taking steps to strengthen children in those areas. Acceptance can include being open to and accepting the child's need to grow and change in some way.

Parents can be mindful of their children by looking past momentary behaviors to see their deeper selves. This perspective includes observing their behavior, expressions, tone of voice, and body language to gather information about children's experiences. A child whose parents take a mindful approach is more likely to freely share their thoughts, feelings, and associations as well—more information for parents to observe. Parents vary in their comfort levels with this kind of observation, but the reward of applying themselves to it is greater attunement and movement toward healthier attachment.

Using a mindful approach, parents can keep in mind simultaneously both the immediate moment and the big picture. Parents can attune to and pace their children while holding an overarching view of their goals as parents. When parents know what they want for their children and their family relationships, they can take steps to move in that direction. They can calmly, nonjudgmentally assess how their children are doing: developmentally on track or off track; troubled in some ways, delightful in others. The goal of mindful parenting is being able to accept children's strengths and weaknesses with love and compassion.

Mindful parents can also nonjudgmentally observe themselves as parents. They can calmly, without shame, look at their behavior with their children. Certainly, most parents will detect areas where they are proud of their parenting and areas where they feel a need to make changes. Noticing and accepting areas of weakness gives them targets to improve. When they are aware of where they want to shift and change, they can thoughtfully, calmly intervene to make it happen.

Providers can hold an accepting and nonjudgmental stance when parents share the ways they are not happy with their parenting and want to change. Parents can feel particularly vulnerable or easily shamed in their roles with their families. As a mindful provider, remember to take time to acknowledge what is going well; focus on recognizing their strengths as parents. Hold the awareness that most parents have good intentions toward their children, and that children do not need perfect parents—they need real parents who try to be attuned, connected, and helpful. Parents being harsh with themselves about their parenting weaknesses is not useful. Being discouraged and angry will only undercut their efforts to shift in a positive direction.

Even as we extol the value of a mindful approach, we recognize that there is no "perfect" in mindful parenting. This focused awareness is not a state that anyone can hold all the time. Our connection to our highest self—the one from which we can parent thoughtfully—will come and go. Parents (and therapists) can aspire to return to that self when they notice that they are off track.

Having a perfect parent will not teach children how to be human and accept their flaws. How painful would it be for a child to be the only imperfect person in the family? How parents handle their own imperfections—ideally, by acknowledging them, making an effort to grow, and moving on—is good modeling for being human. So parents should strive to accept that they and their children are imperfect; they can prioritize compassion and self-regulation; and when they lose it, they can get back on track as soon as possible. Acknowledge, apologize, reconnect, and move on.

It is critical for parents to recognize the limits of their control over their children. As they no doubt already know, they cannot control the members of their families. Even with small children, parents can persuade and influence them, but ultimately their children decide what they will do from moment to moment. What parents can do is determine how they want to think about and react to their children, even when they dislike their decisions.

As Alphonse Karr (1853) wrote in *Lettres écrites de mon jardin* (Letters written from my garden; contribution by an anonymous source):

> *Let us try to see things from their better side:*
> *You complain about seeing thorny rose bushes;*
> *Me, I rejoice and give thanks to the gods*
> *That thorns have roses.*

MINDFULNESS IN HEALING PAST ATTACHMENT DISRUPTIONS

While the skills of mindful parenting promote secure connections with children, for children with parent–child attachment issues, this conscious awareness is essential. Children with early attachment disruptions can push more intensely and persistently for negative engagement. For some, this is a way of avoiding emotional intimacy; for others, it is a way to test and ascertain the stability and safety of the parent. Sadly, for some children, negative engagement is the only intimate emotional connection that feels familiar to them. These children may never have experienced thoughtful and patient care before. They may be accustomed to impulsive, emotion-driven, or disconnected adults. So, parents' efforts to be mindfully present are odd and new, and they may react with resistance and testing.

In all of these cases, rather than backing away from the skills of mindful parenting—parenting that is accepting, present, high on positives, and very low on negativity—parents can be encouraged to lean more deeply into these skills. The testing that often occurs is responded to as a cue to more tightly weave the 3 Stands together; to increase one's commitment to adhering to them; and working to return to them following any slip into negativity. Rather than backing off in the face of resistance, parents double down and work to vigilantly energize any positives they see in their children and to recognize any glimmer of success. They can pour on the attention, animation, and enthusiasm. Therapists can coach these parents to energize children freely and warmly while doing their best to decrease energy toward problem behavior. Self-awareness and mindfulness are required to engage in this process, and therapists can support parents in noticing where they have become more reactive and less mindful and in turning back toward the kind of engagement that promotes earned secure attachment.

When children are acting out in any way, no matter how large or small, caregivers should contain their energy: say little, emote less, do all they can to appear relaxed and soft in terms of body language and expression. Parents can take acting out as a cue to step back and breathe to bring their bodies and minds to a calm state. While doing so, they should remain poised to pounce on any hint of a turnaround they can find: any decrease in acting out, any effort to get back on track, or even a behavior they don't like, but that is less terrible than usual.

This mindful approach to acting out is enacted in the family context of clear rules that, when followed, are celebrated loudly and clearly and with enthusiasm. Dealing with broken rules is discussed in depth in Part IV. For now, parents should set limits reliably and with as little passion as possible.

All of this is a big ask. Mindfulness, thoughtfulness, and self-control require a great deal of effort. The job of the therapist is to keep the focus on the 3 Stands and to provide a positive and optimistic stance, highlighting parents' and children's efforts and successes, no matter how small.

Practice Is Key

Any habit becomes stronger through practice. As described earlier, our brains lay down pathways that are reinforced by repetition, so when parents practice being calm and patient, they build their ability to return to calm during a time of agitation. What parents practice, they are more likely to repeat in the future. Just as we develop an automatic ability to play an instrument through practice, practicing responding to children in this way leads to its becoming automatic and second nature over time. As any successful musician knows, it takes years to develop ease and facility with the foundational skills of playing an instrument—and maintaining them requires ongoing practice.

Some individuals find self-reflection easy, while others do not—based, perhaps, on their past experiences, neurobiology, or current living situations. For example, if parents' home lives are calm and they are treated with kindness, it is natural that they would feel safe and interact thoughtfully with others. However, if they are surrounded by criticism or tension, they may need to purposefully create a state of emotional presence and acceptance in order to self-reflect. In the latter situation, more practice of simple conscious awareness, noticing and feeling emotions, and responding rather than impulsively reacting will be needed for the building of mindful parenting skills.

SPECIFIC SITUATIONS: FOCUS ON THE ATTACHMENT RELATIONSHIP

In working with children and families, there are some circumstances where a direct focus on the attachment relationship is needed for successful treatment. In these cases, the interventions should be preferentially channeled through the parent–child relationship, not the therapist–child relationship.

We recommend this approach with children who struggle with high intensity, trauma, loss, or negative identity; or in situations involving divorce or adoption. Therapists in these situations should remain aware that the attachment relationship with parents is the conduit to effective intervention. A few of these areas are discussed below.

Correcting a Negative or Self-Destructive Identity

When children have severe problems with identity, see themselves as bad, they may identify with being broken, unlikable, ill-behaved, a failure, dumb, or boring. In more extreme cases, these kids sometimes identify with being evil or aligned with the dark side of life. They may be fascinated by blood, fire, and gore, becoming overly excited about violence in media or play. They may show a lack of remorse or conscience, behave in ways that are cruel or destructive, or sabotage their own success.

Keep in mind that children's narratives about their lives link their experiences together and lie at the root of their view of themselves. These narratives are also at the heart of extreme negative self-views. A positive story and a negative story serve the same purpose: organizing and making sense of one's own life—making it appear consistent and logical. For the therapist, breaking into a client's negative self-story can be challenging, because that story is both purposeful and self-perpetuating. In less extreme cases, an effective way to do this is to provide them with honest, undeniable positive feedback that can shift the narrative in a positive direction. In more extreme cases, the strategy is the same, but it will require more effort and time to change identity in a positive direction. This approach often means more patience on the part of adults and children, more creativity in seeking out and communicating positives, and high levels of emotional support or scaffolding to support those who feel very wary and vulnerable in the process of change.

When a family sets the goal of positively influencing a child's identity, a good place for the therapist to begin is by helping parents raise their awareness of the voice they use in interacting with the child. This can be a turning point for some parents. Parents communicate with their children almost constantly. It is useful to notice whether they are yelling, correcting, or expressing pride. Parents may find valuable insights simply by being curious about their style of communication. It is worth the time to explore how the tone of parental attention serves to reinforce a child's behavior and self-identity. Often parents are surprised to notice the degree to which it is natural to speak up about a child's errors and misbehavior and remain silent about his successes and assets. When adults tell children that what they did was terrific, the children file it away. Over time, and with multiple bits of accurate feedback about their successes, a new identity can gradually take over and replace a negative one.

To build a positive identity, parents can start by choosing to expend energy by pointing out children's success, supporting the choices they make in the right direction—not with empty praise, but with specific facts that children can add to their growing notion of who they are. Our goal is to augment the child's self-talk to include notions such as: "I am a creative problem-solver." "I am fearless in stating my needs." "I can express anger without hurting anybody." Even when a problem occurs, the focus can quickly shift back to success, and the error is instantly in the past; what is essential is now—a now in which the child is not hitting.

This shift in energy requires parents to exercise self-awareness and self-control. At the moment children are misbehaving, it is very tempting to focus on the misbehavior, talk about it, maybe even yell about it. But this approach only serves to reinforce to children how bad they are. Instead, providers can recommend parents use self-control and calmly say "no" to the misbehavior. Then they can use all their pent-up emotions and parenting energy to anticipate the next moment when they can point out who children really are: wonderful kids with growing wonderful behavior.

IDENTIFYING WITH AWESOMENESS: CASE EXAMPLE

I once worked with a little girl who lacked self-confidence. She felt inadequate and incompetent, tending to assume her decisions were wrong.

Her parents worked hard to build her up, pointing out to her the small successes she was having several times a day. They commonly made comments such as, "It is awesome that you finished your homework"; "You are so generous to have helped your brother"; and "I love your cooperative attitude—you came the first time I called."

As accurate and unrelenting positive feedback added up, she

started to internalize positive messages about herself. One day she asked, "Dr. Sylvester, does everyone have awesomeness like me?" When I answered yes, she smiled and said, "I thought so!"

E. S.

Childcare Choices: Day Care and Attachment

All adults who serve as caregivers in children's lives play a role in shaping their development. For this reason, parents should ensure that all significant adults in their children's lives have elements of security embedded in their caregiving, and can fortify—or, at least, not work against—the therapeutic steps being taken on behalf of the children and family. In exploring child-care options, therapists can encourage parents to use the basic elements of security to help ensure a rich and supportive environment, including open emotional communication, clear and consistent rules, and a safe place to make mistakes and learn.

A review of the literature shows that studies have reported clearly conflicting results about day care. It has been found to both increase and decrease behavior problems, and to have no effect on behavior problems; to have positive, negative, and negligible impact on cognitive development; and to benefit, negatively impact, and fail to impact the parent–child relationship. The confounding factor appears to be the quality of the childcare. There are so many facets of care that children react to that it is tough to compare one situation to another.

The quality and quantity of children's day care can affect them cognitively, emotionally, and socially. One study examined both the quality and quantity of day care with 1,364 children from ages birth to 4 and a half years old (Vandell et al., 2010). They later evaluated the children's functioning at age 15. The results indicated that higher quality and lower quantity of day care predict better cognitive performance and academic achievement. These qualities are also predictive of lower propensity to misbehave, take dangerous risks, and behave impulsively in adolescence. More hours of care, however, predicted greater risk taking and impulsivity at age 15. Furthermore, it appears that when the quality of care is high, day care is not excessively stressful and can be beneficial for children.

Most children are quite tolerant of being cared for by multiple people and can grow and thrive whether cared for primarily at home or through a blend of home and high-quality childcare. Some specific indicators of attachment-sound day care include caretakers who do the following (including elements of the 7 essential attachment needs):

ATTACHMENT-SOUND DAY CARE QUALITIES

- Maintain a safe environment with secure adult supervision
- Maintain an age-appropriate child-to-adult ratio (see below)
- Take sincere interest in the children
- Display a warm and affectionate attitude
- Answer children's questions patiently
- Get down to the children's level to communicate
- Listen to the children
- Talk about feelings
- Reliably comfort an upset child
- Focus more on engagement with children than on chores and other duties
- Make respectful physical contact with the children
- Create stable and consistent environments
- Show up reliably as key caregivers
- Spend group and individual time with the children
- Retain playfulness
- Have age-appropriate activities, toys, and games
- Have clear expectations, set clear limits, and follow through consistently
- Offer positive reinforcement and praise specifically
- Correct behaviors without harshness or criticism of the child as a person

Instinctively, parents are often anxious about making childcare choices. Parents wonder what type of day care to use, how many hours of care are optimal, what adult-to-child ratio is acceptable, and what the effects of childcare might be, for better and for worse. Much research has been conducted on the impact of day care on infants and preschoolers. Unfortunately, these studies are highly contradictory.

The National Institute of Child Health recommends that infants 6 to 18 months be enrolled in an environment with a 3:1 child-to-adult ratio. When seeking childcare, parents should look for centers with an adequate staff-to-child ratio and a stable caregiver staff with low turnover. As a rule of thumb, inferior-quality childcare, higher child-to-adult ratios, and longer hours in day care correlate with more adjustment difficulties and other problems in children. Of course, more sensitive children are even more affected by the quality of their day care experience.

Ultimately, the current state of our knowledge affirms that the effects of parenting far outweigh the impact of day care quality, and that when the parents' choice is congruent with what the parents believe is best, it works out better for the children.

Divorce and Visitation: Attachment Security

It is a common occurrence for children to be raised in blended families, with parents and stepparents. While adding new parental figures into the most intimate spheres of children's lives is often initially uncomfortable, it is also often successful. Stepparents can be a part of the larger village that humans have always relied upon to raise children well.

As the transition to a blended family occurs, adults must take responsibility for making sure the transition is successful. This is not a job for the children. It is incumbent on birth parents to interact positively with one another and with stepparents. Birth parents have the power to model healthy acceptance of the new family structure. They can, through their actions and words, frame the new family constellation as acceptable, secure, and healthy.

Some children take such transitions in stride, while others need time to grieve the loss of their original family structure. They may express their feelings of loss with anger, anxiety, sadness, or misbehavior. While birth parents should set appropriate limits for misconduct, sensitivity and acceptance of children's emotions about their changing lives is critical.

Stepparents have a different job altogether. They face the challenge of building a relationship with children they do not know well, and who do not know them well. Stepchildren can be reluctant or guarded in forming a connection. Their stepparents' primary job is to focus on being available but not intrusive, being trustworthy and fun, showing interest in the children and not just the new partner, and allowing the depth of connection to be defined by what children find comfortable. Only gradually, after earning trust, can stepparents effectively set limits with their stepchildren.

It may not be satisfying for parents to set aside a new romance to focus on parenting; however, it is the adults' responsibility to prioritize the children's feelings and developmental needs. Children need to feel that they are the priority of their primary parents, regardless of family changes. This helps them to stay on the path to healthy development.

The following list offers a resource for therapists working with parents in the process of divorce. Providers can use this to guide their work with the families in their practice or can share the guide with them directly. These guidelines are supportive of attachment relationships during and after divorce and give the step-relationship a good chance of thriving. These are suggestions that all caregivers can follow.

CHEAT SHEET FOR PARENTS AFTER DIVORCE

Do not:

- **Introduce new dating partners to children** soon after a separation. Protect children from having to meet people when parents are in casual dating relationships. It is stressful for them to meet new people, have to decide if they like them, wonder about a future together, and then see them go away, repeatedly.
- **Communicate with the other parent via the children.** This applies

for minor topics like visitation logistics but is especially true for major topics like a parent's remarriage plans. If a parent is remarrying, the ex-partner should hear it from the parent, not the children.

- **Ask the children to keep secrets** from other parents.
- **Place new stepparents in a position of setting limits with stepchildren.** After the positive aspects of the relationship are in place, limit setting can gradually be introduced for young children. For children who are older when the stepparent is introduced, limit setting may always be the responsibility of the primary parent.

Do:

- **Gradually introduce a new relationship partner to the children** only when that relationship seems likely to be permanent.
- **Be clear with the children that the new partner will not replace** the primary parent. The connection will be different and (hopefully) fun and supportive.
- **Allow the children to like and enjoy a stepparent,** even if the parent has other feelings and opinions about the person.
- **Allow children loyalty to all parents.** Do not ask children to take sides in a conflict between parents; do not ask children who they want to live with or who they like best.
- **Allow children to have negative feelings** in response to the changes in their lives, including the addition of stepparents. Set the limit at rude behavior, not angry or sad emotions.

Adoption: Meeting a Child Later in Life

There are many different ways in which children come to live with their parents, including birth, stepfamilies, and adoption. Unlike parents who raise their children from birth, some people raise children with established parent–child attachment patterns from prior caregiving relationships.

Children with previous secure attachment relationship are typically capable of transferring this attachment pattern to their new parents. They may need to grieve the loss of their prior caregivers, but fortunately have the foundation needed to connect in a meaningful and healthy way.

However, many children have had a rocky start and will transfer a disrupted attachment pattern into the new parent–child relationship. This disruption can take place even if the initial caretaker was physically present and safe but was emotionally unstable. As discussed above, disrupted attachments also arise from the loss of a primary parent due to death, abandonment, severe illness, mental illness, or lengthy separations. Moving through the care of many people (grandparents, family friends, babysitters, nannies) can also create attachment difficulties. These early experiences set up a premature awareness that there are no guarantees of relational stability in life, which can affect children's ability to connect with and trust others later on.

When children experience neglect or abuse, more severe relational disturbances occur. These children do not enter interactions with new adults with a sense of safety. Abuse and neglect interrupt children's budding sense of trust that a caring, responsive caretaker is available. In these cases, children develop defenses against trusting adults—defenses that take root at the neurobiological level.

In parenting these children, it is necessary to address their grief and trauma and to rework their attachment relationship patterns, which were created in dysfunctional relationships and are no longer adaptive. Specific clinical guidance for working with adoptive families can be found in Dan Hughes's work including *Attachment-Focused Family Therapy* and its companion workbook (Hughes, 2007, 2011).

Remember, our attachment relationship patterns are literally built into our brains. Merely interacting warmly and in attunement with a child who has a history of caretaker loss, neglect, or abuse cannot quickly change this pattern. Only time and the ongoing experience of therapeutic parenting can gradually and incrementally alter it. Parents addressing attachment disruptions can be guided to work with great patience, persistence, and consistency to connect in a safe and reliable way. Repair from a history of trauma or loss is a slow and continuous process, and every movement toward health is invaluable (see Part III, Emotion, Stress, and Regulation).

HEALING STORIES AFTER ATTACHMENT DISRUPTIONS: LIFE BOOKS

In therapy, life books can be invaluable in the process of reworking a child's life and personal narrative—particularly a life that has included early disruptions. This book is constructed with the child and directed by the child. Life books are essentially chronologically organized scrapbooks that lay out the important people, places, and experiences of a child's life in words and pictures. They may include summary statements articulating what the child saw or felt, who they lived with, why the child was where they were, or why they left that place. A life book can include art, photographs, drawings, or letters, or whatever the child considers valuable or representative.

A hint to therapists: Often, adopted children have no pictures of early caretakers or homes. You can still create a life book using the child's drawings, images of animal families, or works of art representing families.

A completed life book is a concrete, balanced representation of the child's life: a life that makes sense, is organized, and explains what has happened so far. These books are useful for creating a mental history with the child that clarifies what the child may have been confused about or can clear up misunderstandings about feeling responsible for adult problems.

A child should not just be presented with a life book that was made by someone else. The child must be involved in the construction of the life book, as it is the construction of the story that is therapeutic.

TOUCH AND SAFE CONNECTION AFTER ATTACHMENT DISRUPTIONS

People often associate touch with feelings of attachment, and children with attachment complications often have issues with touch, either avoiding contact or being unusually clingy. This behavior is an outgrowth of their insecurity in relationships, manifested by either wanting to avoid connection and touch—which they worry will be painful—or clinging to a caregiver in a desperate attempt to gain security or control.

For an avoidant child, therapists can encourage parents to gradually add low-stress touch such as fancy handshakes, high fives, brief pats, or thumb wrestling. Games that involve occasional contact are a lower-stress way to introduce and desensitize touch for a touch-aversive child. Parents can acclimate children to safe touch by gently challenging the children's preferred distance by settling in a bit closer. This pacing requires parental sensitivity to find a form of touch that the children enjoy and can accept as loving and not threatening. Parents should avoid tickling or forced contact.

When children use touch excessively, it is often interpreted as neediness, but that is not always the case. Overtouching can grow from the children's search for an attachment figure or from not learning appropriate physical boundaries. It can also be a means of controlling social interactions. For children who demand touch and are always in contact with parents or making affectionate contact with strangers, increasing boundaries around touch is an important goal. It is valuable to teach children that both people must want touch. Parents can articulate to children that they now have a loving family, and they can learn to get their touch needs met in the family. Some families find it useful to discuss how touch is done differently now that the child "is a family boy" or a "family girl."

For more in-depth interventions, Theraplay activities are often useful for building positive associations to touch (Booth & Jernberg, 2009). Over time, these activities can build up to a "snuggle and touch time." A very useful intervention for working through attachment issues is *Core Attachment Therapy*, developed by Dorothy Derapelian (2015), LCMHC. This child-centered form of family therapy reworks early attachment experiences through structured parent–child games and activities. We have found it to have a powerful and lasting effect.

CONCLUSION: IT'S ALL ABOUT ATTACHMENT

Common sense and research concur: It's all about attachment. The quality of the attachment experience in early childhood lays the neurobiological groundwork for many of the basic features a person then carries across life. Relationship success in childhood and beyond, feelings of safety and security across life, ability to self-regulate, and self-image are all outcomes of early attachment relationships. Given the profound importance of this early connection, it is incumbent on family therapists to be attentive to the quality of the parent–child interactions being experienced by their little patients and to intervene at this level whenever possible. Our work begins with taking into account the attachment status of the parents and their ability to read and meet their children's attachment needs.

Our approach to relationship-based parenting begins with therapists creating a safe environment for parents and children. Attunement, stability, pacing, warmth, responsiveness—which, not coincidentally, mirror the features of an early stable attachment relationship—are the building blocks of a therapeutic relationship. In this context, therapists are able to enter the world of the family to help shift relational patterns.

We recommend beginning therapeutic work with the parents alone, focusing on psychoeducation and building skills in relationship-based parenting and mindfulness. As parents refine their parenting style, they will be increasingly able to meet their children's 7 essential attachment needs with consistency, sensitivity, and accuracy. Emotion self-regulation on the part of the parents is a critical aspect of this work, as it links to the attachment system at a neurobiological level. As parents build their capacity, children follow along. This is the focus of Part III, Emotion, Stress, and Regulation.

PART III

EMOTION, STRESS, AND REGULATION

When children feel understood, their loneliness and hurt diminish. When children are understood, their love for their parent is deepened. A parent's sympathy serves as emotional first aid for bruised feelings. When we genuinely acknowledge a child's plight and voice her disappointment, she often gathers the strength to face reality.

HAIM GINOTT, ALICE GINOTT, & WALLACE GODARD,
BETWEEN PARENT AND CHILD

7

Orientation to Theory and Science: Family Emotions

Our emotional development, like our attachment development, is based on our neurobiology and bolstered by healthy parent–child relationships. Children have varying emotional makeups from birth, and each child's neurobiological substrate is unique. The passionate child is likely to remain passionate, the sensitive child sensitive. However, this base system is always modified by experience, particularly early experience in the family. Parents' responses to their child's emotions, their willingness to comfort, their acceptance or judgment of the child's experience, and their tendency to escalate, dismiss, or attune are taken in by the child and modify the child's innate emotional system. When things are going well in the family, the child feels their emotional experiences are acknowledged and respected and that help is available if needed.

If problems arise in the emotional system, we propose using the parent–child relationship as an entry point for treatment interventions. Assisting parents in shifting to more attachment-sound, neurobiologically sound parenting practices serves three goals. First, these practices are more effective in helping a child learn to manage their own innate, neurobiologically based temperament and emotional style; second, they help create safety for the child; and third, they help to heal any maladaptive patterns that have been built up in the family system.

EMOTION REGULATION

Emotion regulation is a term used to describe an individual's ability to modify or soothe their inner emotional experiences and control their emotional responses. It helps us turn the intensity up or down, or shorten or lengthen the duration of our emotions. For example, a person might attempt to manage grief after a friend moves away through a distraction, such as watching a movie, which can help reduce sadness at the moment but does not resolve the underlying feelings. Alternatively, the person might use cognitive tools to reduce their grief by reevaluating their situation and recalling that they will see their friend online next week. Or, they may self-soothe with the reassurances that they will feel better over time and visit with other friends. Mindfulness practice is another path to self-regulation, which can lower reactivity to painful emotions overall. Emotion regulation can also be utilized to assist in meeting a goal. For example, a parent may be feeling anxious about a deadline at work, but their immediate goal is to help their child with their bedtime routine. The parent can utilize emotional regulation skills to manage their feelings and focus on their intended goal of helping their child. Goal-focused emotion regulation helps a person complete a task by lessening emotional distraction, increasing mental focus, and managing frustration to achieve the end goal (Gross, 2014; Gyurak & Etkin, 2014).

Emotional regulation is a key focus for the family therapist, and it begins by bolstering parental self-regulation. A sensitive and adaptive home environment is where children begin to learn about their emotions and how to manage them. When children have emotionally aware and responsive parents, they will eventually learn to regulate their own emotions (Thompson, 2014).

Children, by nature, are emotionally and physically reactive. They react passionately and often overflow with unbridled feelings, both positive and negative. Their abundant emotionality and physical expressiveness can both delight and provoke the adults around them. As children's nervous systems are not mature enough to manage intense emotions or social conflicts, they need stable, mature adults to help them learn to adapt and cope with stress. They cannot yet regulate themselves autonomously.

At times, parents can feel overwhelmed by the raw emotional expression, constant demands, and ups and downs of raising children. Parents can be flooded by the cries of a baby, exasperated or aggravated by the acting out of a 2-year-old, or offended by the irrational rejection of a teenager. Here is where family therapists come in: They bring a buffer to help regulate a stressed family system. When parents or caregivers cannot find their emotional stability, it is hard for them to manage the chaotic emotions of children. A dysregulated adult is incapable of appropriately supporting a dysregulated child. An informed therapist can offer developmental information to calm parents' fears and teach parenting skills to help with conflict and behavior problems.

Most important, however, is the emotional support and regulation that the therapist brings to the whole family. A provider's stability, presence, and emotion management offer a port in the storm. Parents who feel understood and soothed by another stable adult can better weather parenting challenges at home. Stress is easier to handle with support. Once parents feel supported, their emotions acknowledged and regulated, they can better guide their children to learn to cope with distress and manage their own emotions.

As discussed in Part II, when children's essential attachment needs are met, a foundation is laid for self-awareness, social development, self-esteem, and self-regulation. This supports healthy development. An outgrowth of a secure parent–child attachment is the ability to regulate emotions. Here in Part III, we focus on the development of children's emotional worlds and their capacity to understand and manage their feelings, and on strategies that support parents in helping children develop emotion regulation.

CHILDREN'S EMOTIONAL INTELLIGENCE

Childhood is ideally an extended time for children to learn to recognize and manage their emotional world. Emotional intelligence (EQ) gives children the confidence to be flexible and resourceful, to revel in joy, and to be able to work through frustration and disappointments—to thrive as unique individuals in a complex world. It is best if they learn these skills in childhood when the brain is primed for learning (Cozolino, 2014; Fonagy et al., 2010; Gross, 2014; Hietanen et al., 2016; Panksepp & Biven, 2012). Although they can develop new skills later in life, it is much easier when they are young.

In developing emotional competence, children also strengthen self-confidence, resilience, and behavioral control. These basic assets of emotional intelligence are at the foundation of most academic and social achievements (Austin et al., 2005; Tough, 2012). Mental intelligence alone cannot bring about accomplishment and life satisfaction. Research has found that emotional intelligence is more predictive of life success than standard IQ (Austin et al., 2005; Bastian et al., 2005; Helliwell, et al., 2017; Palmer et al., 2002).

Children rely on their parents and caregivers to help them cope with difficult emotions and organize themselves to resolve conflicts. As we have discussed previously, a secure parent–child relationship serves as a buffer to intense adversity and guides children to find creative ways to resolve problems or cope with hardships. In this way, caregivers provide children the footing needed to develop self-awareness, emotional resilience, and confidence (Middlebrooks & Audage, 2008).

Eventually, children mature and internalize what they have learned from their caregivers. They learn to manage their own emotions and confidently make good decisions, even when under stress. As they experience and learn to manage their feelings in different settings, they develop psychological flexibility.

Play and joy are also essential emotions to share with children. Although we may focus on coping with negative emotions, joining children in positivity is critical to developing a full range of healthy emotional intelligence. As Allan Schore (2012) states, "Affect regulation is not just the reduction of affective intensity, or the dampening of negative emotion. It also involves an amplification, an intensification of positive emotion; this condition is necessary for more complex self-organization" (p. 229).

WHAT ARE EMOTIONS?

Most people recognize their emotions and make personal decisions based on them. Nevertheless, emotions are difficult to define. Humans label emotions based on past experience and context; these labels become mental constructs that are linked to internal states.

For example, infants may feel warm and nurtured around their parents. Eventually, children will associate labels with their emotional experiences: *satisfied, cared for, safe.* These positive emotions become part of their repertoire and link to the experience of feeling satisfied while being with their parents. However, when they are fatigued and fussy, children will have a very different experience. These emotions gain their own labels, such as *tired* or *irritable*, which they will come to link to that inner experience. Of course, this is a theoretical description, but it describes what we do know about emotional development (Hietanen et al., 2016; Nummenmaa et al., 2014; Porges, 2011; Siegel, 2012, 2020).

According to Dan Siegel (2012), "Emotion is a commonly used word in everyday language, yet it surprisingly does not have a commonly accepted definition." In interpersonal neurobiology, emotion is defined as an integrated process that links people's internal biochemical states with their external and social experiences. To the individual, the feeling is inextricably linked to the experience.

Although scientists from different disciplines define emotion from different perspectives, they generally agree that emotion is a mental state or process in which a person: (1) experiences an event (an internal or external stimulus), (2) has a neurophysiological response to it, and (3) develops a mental representation of that experience (a thought or feeling). Said another way: Stimulus leads to neurophysiological response; mental representation is created; and impact is experienced and expressed as an action or thought. This mental process is recursive and can alter the emotional experience; it can cycle back to change or reinforce the initial emotional response.

Emotions are not fixed and do not reside in one place in the body. They are the result of a person's continually changing neurobiological processes interacting with their internal and external experiences, which then alters their nervous system and physiology (Byrne, 2019; Gross, 2014; Hietanen et al., 2016; Panksepp & Biven, 2012; Siegel, 2017). As an example, a person may hear the sound of someone yelling (stimulus), experience an acceleration in their heart rate (physical response), and then feel fearful (emotion). Later, they may discover that the original yelling was actually a display of joy, which may then reduce their heart rate and shift emotions to relief or perhaps happiness. Emotions can be complicated and mercurial. They create a transient state of mind that triggers an internal response and influences subsequent interactions.

Although each individual defines their emotional world on a personal level, research suggests that there are universal categories of emotional experiences and expressions that exist across cultures, such as sadness, anger, joy, surprise, fear, and disgust (Table 7.1). These shared emotions are considered by scientists to be a way of categorizing familiar social and neurophysiological experiences (Darwin, 1899/2011; Hietanen et al., 2016; Nummenmaa et al., 2014; Panksepp & Biven, 2012; Siegel, 2020). Learning to identify one's emotions is comparable to the development of an internal language, and it is required for the development of emotional awareness and regulation.

People can start to identify their emotions early in life; their culture and family experiences color the process. As children mature, they learn to label familiar emotional patterns and regulate their responses based on past

Table 7.1 UNIVERSAL EMOTIONS	
Joy	A feeling of great pleasure and happiness
Surprise	An unexpected or astonishing event, fact, or thing causes mild astonishment or shock
Sadness	A feeling of unhappiness or grief; sorrow or mournfulness
Fear	An unpleasant emotion caused by the belief that someone or something is dangerous, likely to cause pain or a threat
Anger	A strong feeling of annoyance, displeasure, or hostility
Disgust	A feeling of revulsion or profound disapproval aroused by something unpleasant or offensive

SOURCE: Darwin, 1899/2011; Hietanen et al., 2016; Nummenmaa et al., 2014; Siegel, 2020

experiences. Past emotional experiences create expectations, which influence future reactions. The maturity of this psychological process is at the foundation of self-awareness and emotional intelligence.

Emotions Versus Feelings

The terms *emotions* and *feelings* are often used interchangeably; however, scientists discuss the differences. In the field of emotion regulation, emotion is defined as a full-bodied experience—tied to physiology, the nervous system, and past experiences—whereas feelings are defined as our inner interpretation of emotions. In this perspective, feelings are a reaction to emotion (Gross, 2014). Fortunately, for treatment purposes, training to help with emotion regulation is also effective for regulating feelings (Berking & Schwarz, 2014).

Colors of Emotion

Emotions are analogous to the colors of the mind. They add dimension and texture to our experiences. They can help us learn, create, and form relationships. Although most scientists believe that emotions start with a simple evaluation of something as good or bad—a primitive impulse to protect us from harm—the process quickly gets more complicated.

Our emotional capacity is built from the bottom up, simple to complex, in patterns that reflect the evolution of the human brain. Primary emotions are rooted in the more primitive, limbic midportion of the brain, which we share with most mammals, while more complex emotions are created in the more advanced cortex, the upper portion of the brain (Byrne, 2019; Darwin, 1899/2011; Panksepp & Biven, 2012; Siegel, 2017, 2020).

Primary emotions are the foundation for more complex emotions. These basic emotions are found across species and include joy, surprise, sadness, fear, anger, and disgust. Primary colors like red, blue, and yellow mix to create more complex colors such as purple and green; similarly, complex emotions are a blending of basic emotions. With the help of the higher brain, intricate feelings such as trust, pride, guilt, and shame are created.

Caregivers who recognize the whole range of colors help children build breadth and width of emotional intelligence.

PARENTS' ROLE IN EMOTIONAL DEVELOPMENT

Therapists can play a pivotal role in guiding parents to work with their children's emotions at home. Parents who offer emotional compassion and scaffolding when children feel distressed serve as a shield against pain and despair. When parents sympathize with their children's unpleasant feelings, children feel less alone. The parents' presence and caring help them to understand and creatively work through their painful emotions. Furthermore, positive emotional sharing—joyous laughter, loving hugs, playful banter—stimulates neuronal growth in areas of the brain responsible for curiosity and learning. It allows children to set up the expectation of relationships where they can seek pleasure and enjoyment. This positive play with parents also acts as a buffer for stress, decreasing the brain's sensitivity to fear, grief, and anxiety. All of this is the heart of parenting.

Research shows that positive, secure parenting induces feelings of comfort and confidence in children. Positive interactions lead to the release of soothing neurotransmitters such as oxytocin and GABA chemicals that serve as a buffer against stress responses (Cozolino, 2014; Fredrickson, 2013; Porges, 2011; Todeschin et al., 2009). On the other hand, harmful parenting creates feelings of sadness and anxiety in children. These negative emotions trigger the release of stress hormones such as adrenaline and cortisol, which can harm children's emotional and physical development (Lester & Sparrow, 2010; Levine, 2015; Schore, 2012; Shonkoff et al., 2012; Wallin, 2007). Stress hormones are explained in greater detail later in this section.

In this rich context of emotional ebb and flow, children take their first lessons on emotional awareness. Their day-to-day experiences of parents' responding to their feelings, welcoming them or ignoring them, encouraging or discouraging them, attuning to them or belittling them, creates in children an underlying sense of themselves as emotional beings. In these lessons, parents teach their children to identify and regulate emotions on two levels, explicit (intentional regulation) and implicit (automatic regulation), both of which are part of a mature emotion regulation system (Gyurak & Etkin, 2014). When parents regulate their emotions and respond to children's feelings with sensitivity and responsiveness, children develop emotional awareness and healthy emotion regulation, both explicitly and implicitly (Gross, 2014; Luerssen & Ayduk, 2014; Shaver & Mikulincer, 2014; Thompson, 2014).

Acceptance of Emotions

Children observe how the adults around them express and manage their emotions. Are feelings expressed freely or withheld? Do parents express some feelings but deny others? Are they a cause for fear, or are they accepted? Children learn to manage their emotional lives and develop skills to manage conflict by observing the adults in their lives. Some parents find it difficult to accept certain emotions due to their own upbringings, their past experiences, and limitations in their own comfort expressing feelings.

We do not all welcome the full spectrum of emotions. Some feelings are harder to cope with than others. Family plays a big role in setting the stage for our experience with feelings, which in turn can influence the development of emotional regulation. Each family has its own way of treating feelings; some express them directly, while others express indirectly or not at all. In some families, certain feelings are encouraged and embraced; others, such as anger, are discouraged or punished.

Culture and gender also play a role in the recognition and integration of particular emotions (Darwin, 1899/2011; Panksepp & Biven, 2012). For example, historically, in Western culture, boys have been discouraged from expressing sadness or crying, while girls have been discouraged from expressing anger. This has had the impact of limiting the ability of people of each gender to embrace and tolerate the full range of emotions.

When children are allowed to explore all of their feelings within a secure parent–child relationship, they develop the sensitivity and skills needed to regulate their emotions and accept emotional expression in others. They can better negotiate to get their needs met while attending to the needs of others. This awareness is what we call emotional intelligence. If some feelings, like sadness or anger, are rejected, ignored, or punished in families, it will be tough for their children to recognize, understand, regulate, and respond to those emotions.

EMOTIONS IN LEARNING

Emotions are inextricably linked to learning and memory. Most people tend to remember events from the past that are associated with strong emotions—positive or negative. Just as emotions can help the brain make sense of experiences, they can direct attention and prioritize information for learning. Strong emotions can facilitate memory; however, traumatic events can overwhelm children and interfere with learning. Children are best primed for learning when they feel safe, cared for, engaged, and curious. They are most receptive to learning from people they trust and enjoy.

Research on emotion regulation and learning indicate that children need to be able to regulate their emotions in order to learn. This regulation helps them to focus their attention on the task and to delay the gratification of other temptations. Studies have found that when parents are more positive and responsive to their children, their children are better able to regulate themselves for learning, whereas when parents display more negativity, their children perform more poorly on these emotion regulation tasks. It is hypothesized that this decline is caused by the high amount of energy children need to expend to cope with the parents' negativity, leaving little energy for productive learning (Luerssen & Ayduk, 2014).

People unknowingly decide what is critical to pay attention to and what is irrelevant through their cognitive and emotional responses to the environment. While you are reading this book, you are automatically focusing on the words on the pages and the ideas presented—probably not so much on the choice of typeface, the color of the background, or the ambient sounds in the room. The more your emotions are stirred by what you are reading, the greater your focus on it is likely to be. This is why an engaging, exciting teacher can make a lesson stick: They naturally pull attention. A dull lecturer can lead students to dismiss or forget the information taught.

Negative emotions can also trigger learning and memory, but not in a positive, integrated way. An upsetting interaction with a teacher can interfere with learning what was intended, and can cause the child to steer clear of the teacher or shut them out from then on.

Therapists can help parents to time their teaching of their children: optimal timing is when the parents are emotionally connected and the child is experiencing positive feelings. They can also help parents recognize that while happy children are ready to learn from valued parents, upset children either will not learn, or will learn something other than the lesson the parents intended. If a parent is angry after a child does not share his toys with a friend, the parent may see the moment as an opportunity to teach about sharing. However, the child is more likely to learn to avoid the situation that made him feel bad than to learn the sharing lesson, or to learn that he is a bad, selfish child who does not share. Fear, shame, and anger all interfere with the child's ability and willingness to learn the intended message (Brazelton & Greenspan, 2001; Langer, 2016; Schore, 2012, 2015; Shonkoff et al., 2012; Sreenivasan, 2017; Teicher et al., 2003, 2016). The process of teaching is discussed further in Part IV.

PARENTS' EMOTIONAL WELLNESS

Parents' first step in taking care of their children's emotional needs is to acknowledge and manage their own internal emotions and needs. It takes mentally healthy parents to help children manage intense feelings and behavioral excesses. This is some of the more difficult work of parenting. When parents feel overwhelmed, anxious, or depressed, it is hard for them to manage the added stress of their children's immature emotional reactions.

Parents may not realize the need to pay attention to and care for themselves as well as their children. They often put others' needs first and neglect their own care without realizing how this ultimately diminishes their ability to support their children. This self-defeating pattern is essential to discuss and work to resolve. When overwhelmed, parents hold less positive energy, have less creativity to help their children, and may need external support to manage their stress (Brazelton & Greenspan, 2001; Lester & Sparrow, 2010; Tronick, 2007; Winnicott, 1964/1992). Research has concluded that healthy lifestyle patterns improve mood, as well as the brain's growth and neuroplasticity (Ang & Gomez-Pinilla, 2007; Fisher et al., 2004; Mesulam, 1999; Petzinger et al., 2015; Stegemoller, 2014; Vance et al., 2010). And, finally, children tend to follow the lead of their parents. This can be an added motivation to parents to set a good example by taking care of themselves.

HEALTHY LIFESTYLE HABITS TO FACILITATE EMOTIONAL WELL-BEING

Good sleep

Healthy nutrition

Aerobic exercise

Learning new things

Play and creative expression (art, music, dance)

Focused mental attention (reading, meditation, prayer)

Building new relationships

Basic healthy behaviors can easily fall off the radar of busy parents; they may have to be reminded of their importance and enticed with the evidence that emotional, physical, and cognitive self-care actually makes them function better in all areas of their lives, including parenting. As they say in the airline business: Put your own oxygen mask on before you help others. Parents need to care for themselves so that they can care for their children.

Emotionally sturdy parents are well positioned to help their children learn how to handle painful emotions. These parents can help their children learn to calm their own fears, grieve their own losses, and express their own anger appropriately. As children go through the stages of upset and reliably recover after receiving comfort and settling, their experiences carry them along a predictable pathway from upset to calm. In accordance with Hebb's rule—neurons that fire together wire together—this path then becomes wired into their nervous systems with repeated experience (see Chapter 2). As they mature, they follow the path to self-soothing more and more independently. Then, miraculously, children begin to use the care they received as a template to offer soothing to others.

8

Ideal Scenarios: Developing Emotional Regulation

A primary goal for children's mental health is to foster acknowledgment and regulation of emotional states across settings: at home, at school, and playing with friends. With support, children can incrementally learn to regulate some feelings up and others down as they make daily emotional and behavioral decisions. However, children are neurobiologically immature and cannot be expected to regulate by themselves.

The term *regulation* is often used in psychology to describe the process of managing emotions and reactivity (Fonagy et al., 2010; Panksepp & Biven, 2012; Porges, 2011; Schore, 2012, 2015; Siegel, 2020). Emotional regulation begins its development in infancy and early childhood with caretakers doing the bulk of the regulation work. The caretaker interfaces with the sympathetic and parasympathetic branches of the autonomic nervous system, which regulate physiological, emotional, and social states, and help the child shift between them.

Children explore emotional coping options and build skills based on what works for them, whether they are adaptive or not. In the throes of a tough emotional state, a child may decide to intentionally help themselves feel better in a few different ways: They might try distracting themselves, playing vigorously, or talking to their mother about their feelings. Another child may find themselves unintentionally withdrawing, changing the subject, or acting out in reaction to negative emotions.

Children develop these patterns through trial and error or learn them from significant people in their lives. As children try various ways to work through their own emotional states, they pay close attention to their effectiveness and continue to use the strategies that work best in the systems in which they find themselves. A child building competence in the area of emotional regulation learns to tolerate uncomfortable feelings and eventually return to a state of calm.

COREGULATION

Coregulation is a process of emotional soothing created within the context of a relationship. One person may soothe the other, as happens when a mother rocks her baby to sleep; or two people might soothe one another by talking together. Touch, sounds, and gaze can all be soothing in a trusting relationship. Being a source of calm for a child is a win-win experience; it offers a safe haven for children and can create a sense of confidence and pride in parents.

The experience of repeatedly being soothed is one of the 7 essential attachment needs of children. When help is reliably available for calming, the experience is gradually integrated into the child. Calmly supporting children helps them develop a strong emotional foundation (Brazelton & Greenspan, 2001; Medina, 2014; Porges, 2011; Porges & Furman, 2012; Schore, 2015) while promoting the release of oxytocin and GABA, hormones that calm our physiological reaction to stress (Cozolino, 2014; Fredrickson, 2013; Porges, 2011).

Although children will ideally learn coping skills from their parents, it is also vital for them to develop independence and find their own solutions to problems as is age-appropriate. Once children are more mature and can resolve their own distress, they may prefer to soothe themselves and may refuse parental attempts to reassure them. This move toward autonomy is developmentally normal and healthy. Coregulation requires caregivers to keep a sensitive balance between helping children when they need it and holding back when they can soothe themselves.

One area of parenting where this balance plays out daily is the dance of putting a baby down to sleep. Pediatrician and educator Dr. T. B. Brazelton recommended that parents help babies learn to rest when tired by putting them down and seeing whether they can help themselves sleep. If the baby cannot calm down to rest in a reasonable time, parents can gently step in to sing or lightly massage the baby to sleep. When these light interventions are not enough to soothe the baby, it may be time to move into more active soothing such as holding, rocking, or bouncing (Brazelton & Sparrow, 2006).

TOUCH, MOVEMENT, AND REGULATION

Children's breathing and heart rate will quiet when close to a calm adult. The more relaxed nervous system of the adult is sensed by the child (heartbeat, breathing, tone of voice) and slows the child's physical pace. Touch can also be soothing and healing when given by a safe and sensitive caretaker (Cozolino, 2014; Field, 2014; Heller, 1997). For example, researchers found that skin-to-skin contact between preterm infants and their parents enhanced vagal maturity (measured by respiratory sinus arrhythmia), which is essential for the infant's ability to regulate physical and emotional states and social behavior (Porges & Furman, 2012). According to neuropsychology and attachment researcher Allan Schore (2012), emotionally responsive touch between the mother and infant in the first year of life also lays the foundation for their secure attachment system.

Secure, fun, physical play with children also creates the basis for children's comfort and joy within their bodies. Play is related to the ability to develop an awareness of when the body needs to move and when it needs to rest. As our society becomes more sedentary, it is particularly critical to keep playful movement on the family agenda. Movement and exercise are essential to overall mental and physical wellness. People are built for movement; it releases stress, builds endurance, and teaches them about feeling their bodies in space (proprioception). Physical play also facilitates greater integration across children's neurological systems: from central to peripheral nervous systems, from right to left hemispheres, and from upper to lower brain regions.

In the process of supporting children's body awareness, parents need to stay sensitive to children's responses to touch or movement. Is it welcomed, or does it feel intrusive? Do they want more or less contact? Being responsive to children's needs lays the foundation for emotional awareness and healthy boundaries. Hugging, light touch, and rough play can all be ways to connect with children when used with sensitivity to their desires and feelings. The child should always have control to slow or stop any physical play.

Mind–body integration begins in contact with others. It is here that children form self-awareness, body acceptance, and nervous system resilience. Safe physical connections with others facilitate children's early sensory integration. Allowing children space and time for physical activity and play with peers also increases social awareness and social skills. They are testing limits socially and learning physical parameters. Healthy peer play serves to teach lessons about sharing, leadership, following, and saying no. They also learn to coordinate and cooperate with others.

SOOTHING WITH TOUCH

When my son was seven years old, he got sick and needed to take medication for a couple of weeks. Unfortunately, he had trouble swallowing the capsules. As he struggled with it, he started feeling more anxious and could not swallow the medication.

I saw he was feeling anxious. I asked if he wanted to sit with me while he took his medicine. He said "yes" and climbed onto my lap. As he sat with me, I consciously slowed my breathing and calmed my nervous system. I hugged him and encouraged him to slow his breath and relax. He was able to calm himself with physical and emotional support. Then he was able to swallow his pill on the first try.

It took him only one more day of sitting with me to help him relax while taking his medicine. After that, he was able to calm himself and take it on his own. This is an example of coregulation promoting self-regulation.

K. S.

EMOTIONAL RESPONSIVENESS AND EMPATHY

Emotional intelligence emerges from the capacity to recognize and express internal emotions. Empathy for others is rooted in this acceptance of one's own feelings, which then can develop into acceptance and responsiveness with others. Such emotional attunement, as you may recall, creates the foundation for secure attachments and builds close and trusting relationships. Children's emotional sensitivity will develop spontaneously in the context of positive, supportive parenting. When caregivers are empathetic to children's feelings, they lay the foundation for children to respond similarly to others (Brazelton & Greenspan, 2001; Brown & Elliott, 2016; Siegel, 2020).

Parental empathy is a calm and responsive focus on children's experiences and feelings without correction, elaboration, or questioning. Empathy does not mean indulging children's hopes or wishes, changing their feelings, solving their problems for them, or even agreeing with them. Instead, it means attentively listening to children, communicating an understanding of their perspective and reaction.

A theory from cognitive science, called theory of mind, describes the ability to reflect on another's mental state and understand that it can be different from our own (Fonagy et al., 2010; Wallin, 2007). This theory is at the root of compassion. By responding thoughtfully to children's emotional lives, we help them develop a theory of mind that will serve them for the rest of their relational lives. Relational empathy has its origins in the attachment system in the first three years of life where—ideally—children's needs are anticipated and accurately met by attentive caregivers. In this intimate connection, children begin to build a sense that others, like them, have feelings and experiences.

When children's feelings are responded to sympathetically, the negative charge attached to their feelings will soften or fade. This comes through the simple act of focusing on and acknowledging the other person's emotions. Interestingly, painful feelings that are not responded to do not typically weaken and dissipate; instead, they tend to either escalate or go underground, where they sit in an unmodulated form to later reappear unbidden and in full force. Adults who take care to acknowledge children's feelings send a strong message that they are valuable, that their feelings matter, that their emotions are understandable and manageable, and that they are accepted. This level of acceptance is in itself comforting and settling.

Notice that we are discussing acknowledging upset feelings, not dwelling on them. The fine line between acceptance and obsessive focus is essential. Obsessive focus is not productive, can be retraumatizing, and can also teach that intimacy is gained through dramatic displays.

TEMPERAMENT AND SENSITIVITY

Temperament is a personality pattern that is unique to an individual. For example, a person may tend to be introverted or extroverted in their social style, which is an aspect of their temperament. Introverts tend to rejuvenate themselves in time alone; they may like time with others, but prefer one friend or small groups over large gatherings. They tend to want time alone to process feelings internally and sustain emotional balance. Extroverts, on the other hand, tend to recharge in social settings. They usually like to be among groups of people. Although they can work through emotions alone, they often prefer to process feelings with others.

Other temperament qualities include activity level, intensity, adaptability, emotionality, impulsivity, approach/withdrawal, persistence, and distractibility. These are believed to be present at birth and stable across life, with some influence from the environment (Chess & Thomas, 1984; McClowry et al., 2008; Medina, 2010).

Window of tolerance is a term introduced by Dan Siegel (1999) to describe the range of arousal that a person finds pleasant or tolerable. It is determined by an integration of past learned experiences and personal temperament that dictates how we respond to various levels of stimulation. When one's experiences are generally within their window of tolerance, they can smoothly manage the demands of their life. Some people have a broad window of tolerance and are comfortable with a variety of levels and types of input, changes, and new situations; they are seen as laid back or unflappable. They adjust fairly easily to, or even enjoy, novelty. They are likely to be open, flexible, and not demanding of others and are likely to react with ease and confidence in most situations, even new or challenging ones.

People with a narrow window of tolerance are more sensitive or reactive. They are likely to prefer a specific level of arousal and may react with boredom, anxiety, insecurity, or agitation to levels of stimulation even slightly out of their preferred range. Their sensitivity can cause them to be reactive to stimuli, perceive more subtle changes, and feel more easily bored, confused, or overwhelmed. They may respond to more stimulating events with caution or react with great intensity, great delight, or great irritation (Ogden et al., 2006; 2020). These more sensitive people may also be observant of details and highly perceptive in their relationships.

Window of Tolerance: Highly Sensitive and High-Intensity Children

The ideal scenario of parenting is not just for easy children. All children can be responded to in ways that optimize their growth and comfort with themselves. Some children are born with more sensitive nervous systems. Individuals with neurological sensitivities, similar to introverted children, are more easily irritated or overstimulated (Kiff et al., 2011) and are likely to have a narrow window of tolerance. Certain fabrics, textures, or tastes can heighten their discomfort. These naturally sensitive children are often reactive to the environment, their emotions, and other people, which makes their experience of stimulation more intense and their preferred level of stimulation lower.

Ideally, parents are patient and supportive with sensitive children, helping them to respect their bodily experiences and develop skills to buffer themselves. They can teach their children to be thoughtful with themselves and to be patient rather than critical or judgmental. This does not mean that sensitive children should be overprotected or oversheltered but that parenting them requires gentle facilitation of their developing self-understanding. These children can develop coping skills to help widen their comfort zone over time (Kagan, 1998). Also, sensitive children may benefit from outside support to help expand their comfort zone, such as physical or occupational therapy.

Finally, a significant subgroup of children who enter our practices crave high levels of arousal. These children seek out and create highly active and stimulating experiences. They are often described as challenging, fun, tiring, creative, and bright—and they are quite uncomfortable when stimulation levels drop below the intense level they prefer. They are prone to boredom and sometimes to neediness or loneliness. When feeling understimulated or disconnected from others, they may engage in behaviors designed to raise the level of action to a more satisfying level. They may create conflict, tease, defy, joke, distract, or engage in any of a number of other tactics to increase arousal.

Again, the patient and supportive parent can help high-intensity children learn to understand and accept their need for intensity. Over time, they can learn to utilize less disruptive ways to stay within their optimal level of arousal. Key to this process is not responding with greater animation when the child is off track. Also, high-intensity children often benefit from having opportunities for high levels of intellectual, physical, creative, and social activity every day.

When parents understand their children's temperaments—both innate and learned aspects—they can respect the child's tendencies and adjust their expectations accordingly. This is particularly important with aspects of temperament that are harder to live with or are less socially or culturally acceptable. Parents can also help children understand themselves and develop coping skills for more challenging moments without instilling shame or a sense of incompetence. As a result, their children will be better equipped to manage well in nonpreferred situations. Their children can eventually learn to take more active control of their experiences, and to cope with discomfort when it does occur, by developing personal coping skills and selecting their level of engagement in different situations. With support and practice, children with a narrow window can expand their range so that it is easier to cope with new situations and frustrations (Ogden et al., 2006; Schore, 2015; Siegel, 2020). This process will help them develop resilience under pressure. The exception to this rule is extreme trauma, which is never within anyone's window of tolerance—an exception we discuss in more detail later in this book.

MINDFULNESS AND EMOTIONAL REGULATION

> Mindfulness is the awareness that arises from paying attention on purpose, in the present moment, and non-judgmentally . . . in the service of wisdom, self-understanding, and recognizing our intrinsic interconnectedness with others and with the world.
>
> JON KABAT-ZINN,
> *MEDITATION IS NOT WHAT YOU THINK*

Emotional regulation is often guided by conscious thought, or mindful awareness. Mindfulness practices involving meditation, movement, music, art, or prayer have been applied for centuries to calm emotions and focus the mind. Studies have shown that mindful practices raise our awareness of feelings, thoughts, and physical experiences, which improves our ability to emotionally regulate and communicate with others (Broad, 2012; Cozolino, 2014; Goodman, 2016; Harrison et al., 2004; Siegel, 2017). Mindfulness practices also reduce vulnerability to negative, painful emotions, and, with practice over time, serve as an emotional buffer for adversity (Berking & Schwarz, 2014; Farb et al., 2014; Germer et al., 2016). In Part II, we observed how mindful parenting can facilitate a secure parent–child relationship. This thoughtful attention also offers children emotional presence, attunement, and safety.

When things are going right in the emotional life of a family, mindfulness often plays a role. A large body of research shows that mindful meditation calms the nervous system, reduces impulsivity, strengthens emotional stability, and improves cognitive focus for parents and children alike (Burke, 2010; Duncan et al., 2009; Farb et al., 2014; Goodman, 2016; Harrison et al., 2004; Kabat-Zinn, 1982; McGreevy, 2011; Singleton et al., 2014; van de Weijer-Bergsma et al., 2012; Wilson, 2013).

There are many ways to practice mindfulness. It might involve a formal meditation practice or simply setting aside time for thoughtful reflection or writing in a journal. Some people prefer a more physical, movement-based path such as mindful walking, yoga, or tai chi—all excellent practices. Whatever mindfulness modality is used, the evidence is clear: the invest-ment of time and effort contributes to the stability of families. We find that mindful awareness is often a part of the ideal scenario.

MINDFULNESS AND THE BRAIN: COMPONENTS OF EMOTION REGULATION

Mindful meditation practices can support emotional regulation, cognitive functioning, and overall well-being. Researchers have discovered concrete changes to the brains of adults who have a regular meditation practice, such as decreased density in the amygdala (reduced emotional reactivity) and increased density in the prefrontal cortex and the hippocampus (improved mood, self-soothing, and learning) (Kabat-Zinn, 1982; Lazar et al., 2005; Lazar, 2016; McGreevy, 2011; Wilson, 2013). Scientists also found increased neuron myelination (efficient mental processing) (Posner et al., 2014).

Research into mindfulness-based stress reduction (MBSR) programs has found that when highly stressed adults practiced meditation for two hours per week for eight weeks, they reported less stress and showed reductions in cortisol levels (Kabat-Zinn et al., 1992; McGreevy, 2011; Wilson, 2013). Some studies have discovered that spending as little as 10 quiet minutes a day writing in a journal or meditating calms the mind and improves aware-ness and emotional presence (Wilson, 2013).

Parents with a reflective practice of their own can more readily help chil-dren learn and practice these skills than those who do not (Burke, 2010; Cozolino, 2014; Schore, 2017). A family that values mindful interactions compounds their benefits throughout the family system.

MINDFUL PATIENCE WITH A TEEN: AN EXAMPLE

When my son was in middle school, I would sometimes feel impatient with his slow pace while doing homework. If I tried to get him to speed up, he got frustrated with me. That was understandable; I knew that it was not good to rush him. And he was comfortable with his own pace, so that was my impulsive reaction.

One day, I caught myself and slowed down my pace. I asked myself, "What really matters here?" I could approach my true goal, which was to help my son find his own strengths, only if I respected his pace and style.

A mindful approach was to notice my own reactivity, remember what I really wanted for him, and respect his boundaries by asking whether he needed anything from me.

K. S.

9

Problem Scenarios: Emotional Dysregulation with Stress, Adversity, and Trauma

Challenging times are to be expected. Coping with them helps people build confidence in their ability to cope with trials in the future. Everyday stressors can usually be managed through straightforward stress management techniques such as positive thinking, taking a walk, or calling on a family member for support. For other stresses, more therapeutic support may be needed. Although coping with stress helps children build emotional resilience, too much stress or high-intensity stress can cause harm.

Allostasis is a term used to describe the adaptive process of coping with stressful situations; *allostatic load* is the wear and tear on the body and brain that comes from chronic or extreme stress (McEwen, 2005). Clients' allostatic load can be assessed based on the total impact of current stressors. The more pressure a person is experiencing at one time, the higher their stress rating. Even when events are deemed positive, like a promotion or a new home, they add to the current level of pressure.

FAMILY STRESSORS: ASSESSING ALLOSTATIC LOAD

Big events: positive and negative

- A new pet
- Academic pressure
- Learning disabilities
- Academic struggles
- Alcohol or drug use
- An accident
- Behavior problems
- Birth of a child
- Change of school
- Changes in work
- Conflict with a friend
- Death in the family
- Extended family conflict
- Financial problems
- Holidays
- Illness/injury
- Loss of a job
- Loss of loved one
- Marital conflict
- Marriage or divorce
- Mistreatment in the home
- Moving or changes in home
- New job
- Sleep disturbance
- Social isolation, loneliness
- Too busy and overscheduled
- Travel
- Victim of crime

MISSING A PARENTAL BUFFER

Research has found that when parents are uncaring or unsupportive of their children it can increase the long-term consequences of stressors those children experience. Parents can play a buffer role for children under stress. Brody et al. (2013) found that if parents were responsive, warm, and supportive with children aged 11–13 years, the children showed less cortisol reactivity at 19; children whose parents were less supportive at ages 11–13 showed greater stress and reactivity at 19. Fortunately, a negative cycle can be reversed. One study found that family interventions to improve parent–child interactions could reduce some of the negative stress and health consequences of early unsupportive parenting (Chen et al., 2018). Animal studies have also found that maternal caregiving behaviors, such as licking and grooming, decrease stress responses in their offspring (Caldji et al., 2000; Todeschin et al., 2009).

Mild or moderate challenges that allow children to learn how to manage feelings and cope with discomfort crop up naturally. However, if children's emotions are not acknowledged by their parents and are not coregulated, children miss the opportunity to learn the emotional skills of adapting in the moment (Farb et al., 2014; Thompson, 2014). If parents are emotionally present and supportive, they can aid children in building these coping skills. When the whole family is under extreme or prolonged stress, however, even the best parents will find it difficult to be supportive. It is easy to lapse into disengagement or hair-trigger reactivity. When parents are available and compassionate, children can learn ways to manage their feelings and reduce tension, which builds confidence.

The daily demands of family life can strain families with limited resources. Perhaps a couple never developed good coping skills, and the addition of children revealed these limitations; or a couple's emotional resources were sufficient before having children but feel inadequate with their expanding family. Either way, family therapists can offer immediate relief—encouraging families to sustain healthy patterns such as daily structure, positive communication, and emotional support.

If parents are overwhelmed, shut down, or otherwise dysregulated, family therapists should focus first on offering support and building coping skills in the adults before addressing deeper issues. The goal is to help parents get back on track as, in the absence of steady emotional support and guidance, children can feel easily overwhelmed. This commonly leads to increased emotional and behavioral issues, which further stresses the family, leading to a negative spiral. Alternatively, some children may learn to ignore their feelings or let their discomfort settle into their bodies, or they may not learn to self-soothe or seek comfort in others. In either case, when parents are not available to help children cope with stress, children's emotional development is adversely affected.

Children will try to soothe themselves even without adult support, but their coping efforts may appear illogical, self-defeating, and regressive. For example, a young student may attempt to avoid a difficult assignment through flight, by running out of the classroom, down the hall, and into the street. A child's aggression, withdrawal, bossiness, or defiance can be understood as other kinds of self-defeating coping attempts. Children will be more successful if they receive caregiver soothing that scaffolds and supports their attempts.

The development of healthy emotion regulation relies on early attachment relationships, as discussed in Part II. The attachment hormone oxytocin works as an antidote to stress and anxiety; it triggers relaxation and assists in the development of positive connections. This hormone is released in the context of safe and caring interactions, including emotional attunement and play. When these relationships are disrupted or lacking, children's coping systems suffer. As emotional challenges increase or adversity is more extreme, the lack of a robust infrastructure will surface as emotional and behavioral problems. On the other hand, one secure adult attachment can buffer stress and aid children in coping with pressure. In some cases, a therapist is that one secure attachment.

PARENT REACTIONS TO STRONG EMOTIONS

Parents' reactions to strong emotions play a role in their children's emotional regulation. If children are expressing intense feelings, they can easily trigger parents' extreme reactions, which can then perpetuate children's distress. Parents' emotional states or temperaments influence how they respond to their children's strong feelings. They can lead parents to respond with great sensitivity or to ignore or overreact.

An essential component of family therapy is fostering safe and stable parenting. This requires the therapist to openly address with parents their ability to manage their feelings and discuss how this builds trust and positive attachment. Parents who do not find a way to be calm when problems occur destabilize their relationship with their children. It is impossible, and not useful, for parents to avoid having strong feelings—even negative ones—when rearing children. The goal is not for parents to always be happy or to fake being happy. Instead, the goal is to foster movement toward being steady; building capacity to self-regulate when emotionally unstabilized; and not allowing painful feelings (their own or their children's) to break the attachment connection.

Everyone has emotions that they are not comfortable experiencing or expressing. Parents often find that they are more comfortable with some of their children's feelings than with others. They may notice that they are very understanding and patient with a sad, hurt, or worried child but have more trouble remaining calm when dealing with an angry child, or vice versa. This pattern offers necessary information for treatment. Ideally, parents learn to be receptive to all of their child's feelings in the same calm way: allowing them, discussing them, and setting appropriate limits around how to express them.

In light of this, parents may need the additional support of individual psychotherapy or other treatment to expand their ability to manage their feelings and stay open to their children's full range of emotions. This focus in therapy is even more relevant when the family is under stress, or when parents are coping with their own emotional distress.

EXAMPLE: PARENTAL SELF-CORRECTION

One day when my daughter was in first grade, I was particularly tired and irritable—not feeling patient. My daughter was happy, but she was running in the house. I asked her once to slow down, and she did not. The next time, I lost my temper and yelled at her. My face was angrier than called for in the situation. She stopped in her tracks, and I saw the happiness melt from her face. She looked sad, near tears.

My mistake: too intense. I caught myself before continuing to yell; I paused and struggled with my feelings of fatigue and frustration, and the shame I felt for losing my temper. Then I took a deep breath and quieted myself. I felt sorry for my intense reaction and wanted to reconnect with my daughter and her joy. I told her I was sorry for yelling at her. "I did not mean to act so angrily. I am calm again," I said.

Her behavior was still an issue, and I addressed that next. "I need you to change your behavior now," I told her, and she quickly responded—first, by smiling and running to me for a big hug, and then by slowing her pace as she skipped across the house.

K. S.

ADVERSITY, TRAUMA, AND POSTTRAUMATIC STRESS DISORDER

Extreme adversity and trauma differ from everyday challenges and frustrations and can have significant consequences in children's lives. Research has found that exposure to severe or chronic adversity, such as under the circumstances described below, can compromise children's developing brains and bodies and persist into adulthood (Brody et al., 2013; Chen et al., 2018; Levendosky et al., 2002; Levine, 2015; Main & Hesse, 1990; Nakazawa, 2015; Shonkoff et al., 2012; Teicher et al., 2003; Todeschin et al., 2009).

The Adverse Childhood Experiences (ACEs) questionnaire is a measure used to estimate a person's level of childhood stress and trauma. In research, a notable relationship has been found between childhood adversity (such as abuse, neglect, domestic violence, losing a parent, or having a mentally ill or addicted parent) and emotional and health consequences in adulthood. Food or housing insecurity, natural disasters, or accidents can also be significant sources of childhood adversity. Studies have found a strong positive correlation between higher scores on the ACEs survey—indicating more stressful experiences—and higher risk of emotional and physical symptoms in adulthood (Merrick et al., 2018). While not all children who experience adversity develop long-term negative symptoms, they do have higher risk. Chronic childhood adversity is related to higher risks of addictive patterns with food, alcohol, or other substances in adolescence and adulthood. One study found that individuals with four or more adverse experiences, as compared to those with none, were five times more likely to become alcoholic, over twice as likely to become obese, and 46 times more likely to become an IV drug user (Nakazawa, 2015). See the Adverse Childhood Experiences study (Centers for Disease Control and Prevention, 2021) for more detailed online information on ACEs and their impact.

Although extreme adversity is never good for children, they can often recover from the suffering it causes with the understanding and support of a compassionate caregiver. Without this type of support, children's emotions are more likely to feel overwhelming, remain unresolved, and develop into symptoms of posttraumatic stress disorder (PTSD).

Acute Stress

The initial reaction to a traumatic event is the *acute stress response*, which can include a variety of sympathetic nervous system (SNS) responses including fight or flight, anxiety, emotional reactivity, and hypervigilance; or it can include downregulated parasympathetic (PNS) responses including fainting, numbness, depression, and dissociative symptoms. In addition, children may avoid reminders of the traumatic event or may experience memory loss or cognitive distortions related to the event.

ACUTE TRAUMA REACTION

Acute Stress

Intrusive thoughts: reliving the event

Heightened reactivity, hypervigilance

Avoiding reminders of the trauma

Emotional Shock

Numbness

Dissociative symptoms

Physical or emotional detachment

Dreamlike state

Memory loss or distortions

Trauma and Posttraumatic Stress

Events are defined as traumatic if an individual (1) experiences an actual or threatened risk of injury or death, or (2) witnesses an actual or threatened risk of injury or death to someone else (particularly, a family member or friend). Statistics indicate that 66% of children experience trauma by the age of 16 years. While most can recover from acute trauma symptoms after several weeks or months, some children will experience an extended trauma reaction, or posttraumatic stress disorder (PTSD).

The risk of developing PTSD increases when trauma is repeated or severe, if children are close to the trauma, or if the trauma involves people injuring other people. Parents' emotional stability and reactions to the traumatic event play a vital role in children's resolution of the traumatic stress reaction (or lack thereof).

SYMPTOMS OF POSTTRAUMATIC STRESS DISORDER (PTSD)

1. Reexperiencing

- Flashbacks
- Nightmares
- Intrusive thoughts

2. Avoidance
    - Dissociation
    - Avoiding trauma reminders
    - Emotional numbness
    - Shutdown
3. Hyperarousal
    - Anxiety and fear
    - Clinginess
    - Extreme emotional reactivity
    - Irritability, anger, negativity
    - Exaggerated startle response
    - Distractibility or hypervigilance
    - Sleep disturbance
4. Negative changes in thoughts or feelings
    - Exaggerated blame of self or others
    - Reduced interest in activities
    - Feeling socially isolated
    - Negative thoughts/feelings
    - Inability to remember trauma events
    - Difficulty experiencing positive emotions

The trauma reaction of PTSD looks different in children of different ages. Children from birth to age five are likely to display disruptions in eating and sleeping, startle more quickly, and show an increase in separation anxiety. They may also seek more attention and reassurance, show new fears or sadness, act more agitated or withdrawn, and fear people who remind them of the event. As children reach school age, symptoms are more clearly representative of the trauma and more easily understood by adults. Children between five and 12 are likely to recreate trauma scenarios in their play, and to show more aggression, controlling behavior, or somatic symptoms (headache, stomachache). They may also be clingy or show diminished confidence and a decline in their school performance. They may be more agitated and vigilant. They may have an altered time map of events where they confuse order or timing of the traumatic event. They can also begin to detect warning signs around them that they fear will create negative circumstances. For some, PTSD symptoms may include suicidal thoughts or behavior. For adolescents (13–17-year-olds), symptoms of PTSD are often a mix of childlike and adult responses. While they may act out and replay trauma events as younger children do, they may also experience flashbacks, intrusive thoughts, nightmares, or memory blocks as adults do. Other symptoms in teens include impulsivity, aggression, lowered self-esteem, feelings of guilt, and difficulty with friendships. They may feel alienated and isolate themselves. At this developmental stage, young people are more vulnerable to running away or turning to alcohol and drugs.

Abuse and Neglect

Victims of childhood abuse and neglect can suffer from an array of posttrauma symptoms. They experience typical PTSD symptoms like reexperiencing, avoidance, and hyperarousal, along with others like shame, self-blame, decreased self-esteem, aggression, dissociation, and self-destructive behavior. Sexually abused children can also show signs of disruptions in their typical path of sexual development or sexually inappropriate behavior. Children often blame themselves for abuse and neglect, intensifying their feelings of isolation, negativity, and helplessness. These kinds of developmental trauma can have far-reaching consequences that may persist into adulthood.

Here are some factors that mental health practitioners can watch for that increase the likelihood of family abuse or neglect. When these are present, therapists can work to address them before abuse or neglect begins.

- Alcohol or drug abuse
- Financial crises/hardship
- Involvement in criminal activity
- Isolation; lack of support network
- Lack of awareness of child development limitations (unrealistic expectations)
- Lack of nurturing the child

- Parent history of maltreatment as a child
- Parental difficulty bonding with newborn
- Untreated mental illness

Childhood abuse and neglect are serious social problems in the United States and across the world. The youngest children are at the highest risk for abuse, although abuse occurs into adolescence (37% of children ages 0–6; 37% of children ages 7–12; 26% of children ages 13–17). In the United States, 4 million reports of child abuse are made each year, involving 7.2 million children. Of these, 3.4 million receive investigation or services, with 700,000 children per year determined to be victims of abuse or neglect. The largest proportion of fatalities due to child abuse (48%) happen to children under the age of 1 year (US Department of Health and Human Services, 2019).

The majority of reported abuse is due to neglect (65%), followed by physical abuse (18%), sexual abuse (10%), and emotional abuse (7%). The majority of perpetrators of abuse are related to the child in some way (parent/caregiver, 40%; nonparent relative, 50%). On the other hand, the majority of child abuse reports are made by a nonrelative or nonneighbor or by professionals who interact with the child or family (teachers, therapists, social workers).

Children who have experienced abuse are at significantly elevated risk for both psychiatric and physical health problems. In fact, abuse is the single greatest contributor to the risk for psychiatric and medical illnesses—greater than any genetic or other environmental factors (Lippard & Nemeroff, 2020). Risk of mood disorder, stroke, addiction, drug abuse, and suicide are all influenced heavily by a history of child abuse.

POSTTRAUMA RISK FACTORS AND BUFFERS

One major risk factor after a traumatic event is lack of reliable and caring adult support. As mentioned above, one secure adult can buffer the harmful influences of adversity. Mental health providers and other support systems can encourage parents to create a family buffer to reduce the cycle of negativity, enhance emotional security, and prevent further mistreatment of children. It is a worthy goal for therapists to work with parents to build safety and support for children at home by bolstering parents' skills at being consistently open to feelings, raising emotional sensitivity, and reducing any additional pressures. Emotional attunement and soothing can help children cope with strong emotions or physical symptoms after trauma. In Chapter 10, under Posttraumatic Stress Recovery, specific treatment approaches are presented for families after trauma.

Therapists working with traumatized children can also reach out beyond parents and children to assess school environment, friendships, and the broader social community. They can work with schools to ensure that undiagnosed or improperly remediated learning disabilities, bullying, or ineffective classroom management strategies are not adding stress or additional layers of trauma. Schools can work with therapists to ensure that children's academic and emotional needs are appropriately met.

Supportive services such as early intervention programs, parent education classes, home nursing care, childcare programs, and abuse prevention programs in schools can also help to prevent abuse and reduce the long-term consequences of childhood adversity (Blair, 2008; Brazelton & Greenspan, 2001; Davidson & McEwen, 2012; Duncan et al., 2009; Lundahl et al., 2006; Shonkoff et al., 2012; van der Put et al., 2018; Vlahovicova et al., 2017; Winnicott, 1964/1992; Wolfson et al., 1992). Information shared with new parents in these programs can reduce stress and strain on new families, supporting them in learning parenting strategies that prevent abuse (such as how to soothe infants who are crying, including education about the dangers of shaking babies).

NEUROLOGICAL COSTS OF ADVERSITY

Chronic or extreme early life adversity can change the brain. Trauma early in life can impair the development of critical structures and their functions such as the prefrontal cortex, limbic system, and dopamine system, all of which are critical to emotional regulation and stress management. Unfortunately, this regulation is exactly what children need to manage stress. When the developing brain is altered by persistent and extreme suffering, children can become more reactive or more easily panicked or enraged, or they may have more difficulty calming after an irritation (Caldji et al., 2000; Hackman et al., 2013; Hutt et al., 2012; Levine, 2015; Nachmias et al., 1996; Nakazawa, 2015; Sapolsky, 2004; Teicher et al., 2003; Vandell et al., 2010; van der Kolk, 2015).

Researchers have found that chronic and extreme childhood stress impairs development of the prefrontal cortex, corpus callosum, and limbic system, as well as interfering with neuronal growth, myelination, and connectivity. This impaired development often leads to a brain-based vulnerability in emotion management, decision making, motivation, social relating, and learning (Badenoch, 2008; Carrion & Wong, 2012; Cozolino, 2014; Davidson & McEwen, 2012; Nachmias et al., 1996; Schore, 2001, 2015; Shonkoff et al., 2012; Siegel, 2020; Teicher et al., 2003, 2016; Todeschin et al., 2009).

The limbic system contains the amygdala and the hippocampus. Both these structures are critical in the stress or fear response system. The amygdala serves as a panic button that recognizes a dangerous situation and triggers the release of stress hormones, which equip the body to pursue safety. Research has found that children who live in safe and secure environments have relatively small amygdalas; where that structure is smaller, there is more calm and adaptiveness in new or distressing situations. The amygdalas of children who live with chronic or extreme adversity tend to have greater volume. While this allows these children to respond more quickly to stress, they are also more reactive to tension and more impulsive in conflict. The hippocampus, which helps children to learn from experience and regulate emotions, has also been found to shrink under intense stress. These combined changes make it difficult for children to adapt and implement effective coping skills. As a result, children from neglectful or violent environments feel more easily overwhelmed, react more easily and more intensely, and have greater difficulty regulating and thinking clearly.

The prefrontal cortex at the forefront of the brain is the seat of executive functioning, including self-awareness, social sensitivity, emotional regulation, attention span, planning abilities, and self-control. As children raised in safe and secure home environments develop these skills, the thickness of their prefrontal cortex is increased, and this aspect of brain development is reflected in the natural development of strong executive functioning skills. However, children raised in highly stressful situations have smaller and less dense prefrontal cortical structures. A weaker prefrontal cortex region is related to increased impulsivity, difficulty planning, trouble with follow-through, and decreased sensitivity to others' emotions.

Most neurons are coated with myelin, which increases the speed and efficiency of nerve impulse transmissions. A safe and responsive home environment optimizes the development of this myelination, which translates into more rapid processing of information. A highly stressful home can decrease myelination, lowering cognitive performance and raising risk-taking or impulsive behavior.

This science emphasizes the need for secure and safe home environments for children to support their early brain development and neural integration. Emotional regulation and well-being depend on these developments. If excessive stress in children's lives continues and safety is not secured, these brain changes can persist into adulthood (Carrion & Wong, 2012; Lester & Sparrow, 2010; Mate, 2010; Ogden et al., 2006; Porges, 2011; Schore, 2001; Teicher et al, 2016; van der Kolk, 2015). Improving the quality of children's day-to-day lives aids in the repair of brain structures and function—and therapy can be a source of support for building physical and emotional security (Baylin & Hughes, 2016; Chen et al., 2018).

PHYSIOLOGICAL COSTS OF ADVERSITY

Extreme adversity can also have a broad and long-lasting impact on development of children's cardiovascular, respiratory, muscular, endocrine, digestive, and immune systems (see Chapter 2).

Trauma triggers children's bodies to shift into survival mode: an innate autonomic response in which they prepare to fight, flee, or shut down to protect themselves. While these automatic responses improve children's chances of survival when under threat, the bodily changes they trigger are intended by nature to be brief, intense reactions to protect them from danger, not zones in which to live long-term. In a chronic state of crisis, the same responses that can save children in the moment can wear on and degrade their brains and bodies.

Recall that in states of high stress, the nervous system is dominated by the SNS, which triggers the release of fight-or-flight stress hormones such as adrenaline and cortisol. These hormones raise heart rate, increase blood sugar, speed up the breath, and prepare the muscles to move. However, where the physiological jolt provided by adrenaline and cortisol is not used to jump into action, the lingering effects of these activating hormones damage the body and mind (Sapolsky, 2004).

The health consequences of chronic stress are far-reaching and can reduce life expectancy by raising risk of heart disease, high blood pressure, and elevated cholesterol (Kiecolt-Glaser et al., 2010; Middlebrooks & Audage, 2008; Naka-zawa, 2015). Specific physiological costs include weight gain, inflammation, reduced immune functioning, and decreased bone density (Ogden et al., 2006; Sapolsky, 2004; Schore, 2001; Teicher et al., 2003; Thoits, 2010; van der Kolk, 2015). Chronic stress can also interfere with normal, healthy development at a cellular and epigenetic level (Blair, 2008; Brody et al., 2010; Epel et al., 2004; Kiecolt-Glaser et al., 2010; Lester & Sparrow, 2010; Shonkoff et al., 2012).

The effects of extreme adversity change the developmental path of the brain and body. To this end, safety and trauma prevention during the developmental years should be a top priority of our society and our government, including funding for early childhood protection against abuse and neglect. Early intervention to prevent trauma is far more efficient than repairing and healing once the damage has been done. And if trauma does occur, swift and targeted posttrauma treatment of children and their families can reduce the level of harm done and begin the healing process.

NEGATIVE CYCLES OF STRESS AND TRAUMA

As described above, chronic stress increases growth in areas of the brain that heighten reactivity (amygdala) and decrease brain growth in regions that are needed to calm anxiety (prefrontal cortex, hippocampus) (Carrion & Wong, 2012; Cozolino, 2014; Sapolsky, 2004; Todeschin et al., 2009; van der Kolk, 2015). Stress-related hormones sensitize the fear response and increase emotional dysregulation and impulsivity. Stress can interfere with learning and memory and increase the risk of anxiety and depression. These consequences cause children to be more reactive and have less capacity for coping with adversity, which then can create a negative recursive anxiety loop where internal or external resources for correction and repair are limited.

Self-protective patterns that develop to cope with current stressful situations are likely to cause trouble in the future. For example, emotional withdrawal or aggressive acting out can help children deal with painful family situations but can be self-defeating in other circumstances. The resulting frustration, sadness, or anger can then become part of a long-term negative cycle.

Survival Brain: Strengths and Vulnerabilities

The human brain is famously plastic, meaning it adapts to survive in whatever circumstances it finds itself. If children are raised in stressful environments, their brains adapt to optimize the likelihood of survival in dangerous or stressful situations. The shaping of physiology and psychology in response to chronic adversity is actually adaptive for those forced to live in unsafe, unstable, and threatening circumstances. People who are survivors are often quick to respond in a crisis and can persevere through greater adversity than those who grew up under less adverse circumstances—although their responses may lack nuance, sensitivity, and diplomacy.

The survival brain's strength is the tendency to react quickly, decisively, and firmly to any perceived threat. However, the survival brain may find moderate or reflective responses less automatic. When a survivor of trauma or adversity feels elevated emotions, there is a tendency to react intensely and immediately—a response that is highly effective when there is a real danger, but that can create very real problems. Intense reactions could escalate the situation, alienate others, or impede resolution. If not checked, the brain and body well adapted to quick response to adversity (the survival brain) can create a negative cycle of conflict, defensiveness, and withdrawal.

The survival brain is not well suited to life in primarily peaceful, stable, and friendly environments. Its architecture can impinge on one's ability to sustain connection and deal with others sensitively. It is often weak on working in harmony with others, maintaining focus, tolerating a slow-paced experience, and being at peace.

Breaking the Survival Brain Cycle

There is hope for parents who are raising children with survival brains, or those who have survival brains themselves. People can learn to understand and manage their brain's style and, over time, to shift patterns to their advantage.

Although brain-based patterns of interaction do not just wash out over time—survival skills are embedded in the brain's neural structure—they can be shifted toward greater flexibility and patience with intentional work. It is possible to increase the capacity to act and respond with more subtlety where situations demand; movement toward social adaptability and emotional regulation can be developed with time and effort. When working with children, this often begins by helping parents shift. While it may feel disheartening to recognize that trauma changes the brain, healing also changes the brain. Remember that neuroplasticity is present throughout our lives. The treatment described in the section on posttraumatic stress recovery lays out ways to foster such change.

If parents were raised in highly stressful or traumatic environments, they might have developed a brain wired for survival. This may reveal itself early in therapy in the form of intense and impulsive responses to the irritants inherent in living with children—negative reactivity based on the parents' own distressing childhood experiences. There is no blame or shame; parents did not choose to create their survival defenses. Our job, as family therapists, is to accept the survival brain's tendencies and learn to work with them, around them, and in spite of them. Parents committed to this growth are doing the requisite work of parenting.

Remember: A survival brain is not broken or inferior. It is the perfect brain to help one survive in dangerous, stressful situations. Healing means learning to function well when life is safe and secure; when others can be trusted; where there is no need to fight to stay alive. Ideally, parents coming from a history of unresolved trauma or adversity will be able to avoid passing on their fight, flight, or shut down tendencies to their children, instead supporting children (and, by association, themselves) in cultivating a brain wired for trust, thoughtfulness, and self-regulation. Even if survival brain patterning has already been passed down to children, intentional and patient therapeutic work can reverse this patterning.

It is essential to find an entry point through which you can help parents learn to parent calmly and effectively, even with a trauma history of their own. Even if parents do not intend to do their own psychotherapy, as a family therapist you are in a prime position to support the parents on behalf of creating stability for their children. Where you can guide them not to pass the trauma brain on to the next generation, the cycle of dysfunction ends.

Discussion of the survival brain and development of parents' compassion for their own reactivity can be a good use of psychotherapy. Creating clarity about the importance of calm and stability in the home can also be useful, as can the development of self-correction strategies and a reset plan for times when the parents are triggered. In some cases, you may want to refer parents for their own individual therapy. It is often helpful to the whole family.

MENTAL HEALTH DISORDERS IN THE FAMILY

When children live in families with untreated mental health disorders, some specific and well-researched effects can occur. Studies have found that parents with untreated depression are less capable of creating positive connections with their children, which can impair children's emotional stability, sense of security, and healthy brain development. If parents are burdened by depression, their children may not experience the full range of positive emotions, including joy and curiosity. Parental depression can also interfere with the development of secure attachment (Easterbrooks et al., 2010; Toth et al., 2006; Tronick, 2007, 2017; Weissman et al., 1984; Whaley et al., 1999).

Children whose parents suffer from anxiety disorders have increased risk of anxiety. Research indicates that children respond to their parents' worries with increased distress and fear. Anxiety can be passed along genetically through inheritance; it can also develop in children if parents model chronic stress and anxiety. Children are very sensitive to their parents' state of mind and can pick up and react to unexpressed distress (Hutt et al., 2012; Nachmias et al., 1996; Weissman, 1984; Whaley, 1999).

Mental illness can include depression and anxiety, as well as more severe disorders such as schizophrenia, bipolar disorder, personality disorders, or substance addiction. Each of these disorders can impact attachment and be disruptive to children's day-to-day lives and the emotional functioning of the family. Family members can react to mental illness with fear, shame, or isolation, and society often responds to it with criticism and discrimination.

If parents have preexisting mental health symptoms, they can be worsened by the stress of a new child or by day-to-day parenting demands. These parents are likely to have difficulty providing the emotional and physical resources to fulfill their children's attachment needs—including consistency and reliability. Untreated mental illness in parents can impact children's emotional development. Severe mental illness often results in unpredictable or chaotic parenting, which interferes with children's ability to build trust in and count on their caregivers. This dynamic negatively impacts the attachment system (Cozolino, 2014; Karen, 1998; Schore, 2012, 2015; Nakazawa, 2015; Lester & Sparrow, 2010; Wallin, 2007).

PREGNANCY AND POSTPARTUM MENTAL HEALTH

Even before birth, the child experiences effects of the mother's emotional system. During pregnancy, if a mother experiences extreme anxiety or adversity, stress hormones can compromise the fetus's developing nervous system. This development can affect the infant's self-regulation system, making it more difficult for them to cope with discomfort early in life (Cozolino, 2014; Huizink et al., 2003; Schore, 2001, 2012; Schetter & Tanner, 2012).

After delivery, new mothers are vulnerable to postpartum depression, anxiety, or even psychosis, which can start days or months after a child is born (Schore, 2017). This time is usually stressful for all the child's caregivers. A newborn does not have a consistent sleep–wake cycle and has an immature nervous system. The resulting stress and sleep disruption for parents often cause emotional dysregulation. It is common for new parents to feel fatigued or overwhelmed at times. Level and persistence of difficulty vary from parent to parent; while some parents resolve their emotional discomfort quickly, others experience intense tension and require professional support.

When a new baby arrives, family therapists can offer emotional support, resources, and useful information to new parents. Home visits and mother-infant groups reduce postpartum depression and anxiety (Heinicke et al., 1999). A robust support system can reduce new parents' risk for mental health concerns and reduce any harmful implications for the baby.

In the early months or even years after a child is born, untreated postpartum depression or anxiety can cause adverse outcomes for the baby's neurological system. This influence is also present at the genetic level. Epigenetics refers to the fact that human genes are flexible in their actions and can be turned on or off by specific experiences. The expression of genes is affected by chronic adversity (Brody et al., 2010; Epel et al., 2004).

Fortunately, research indicates that acknowledging and treating emotional disturbances during pregnancy and postpartum benefits both mothers and babies. Positive social, emotional, and physical support for women during pregnancy can reduce stress hormones and improve emotional resilience. When mothers feel well supported in their relationships, it reduces felt stress. Also, when women take good care of themselves, they are better able to support their baby's developing body, brain, and nervous system (Paddock, 2016; Singleton et al., 2014; Wilson, 2013; Wolfson et al., 1992).

And maternal self-care, such as maintaining a healthy diet, exercise, and mindful meditation, strengthen both mother's and baby's emotional and neurobiological systems (Paddock, 2016). One study found that prenatal and postpartum massage reduces stress responses, increasing feelings of well-being and promoting neurological growth for both mother and baby (Field et al., 2009; Whiteman, 2017).

IMPORTANT ROLE OF THE FAMILY THERAPIST

Family therapists face the challenge of detecting and intervening when parental emotional disturbance creates an overly stressful, or even abusive, family environment for their children. Therapists are probably well aware that Child Protective Services often cannot intervene for more subtle forms of neglect and mistreatment, although these situations cause chronic and severe stress to many children. Even if therapists identify family safety concerns, their capacity to quickly treat them is severely limited in the cases of personality (Axis II) disorders or other mental illnesses that are less responsive to quick treatment.

The best that therapists can do to fill this crack in the system: Quickly identify at-risk parents, compassionately reach out and build relationships with the family system, and provide the best safety net possible to meet the needs of the family. This process requires attentive management of the impaired parent, with the goal of harm reduction.

When a parent is suffering or depleted, it affects everyone in the family. The good news is that the treatment of mental distress and postpartum emotional disturbance works. Treatment can reduce symptoms, improve parent functioning, and decrease the negative consequences for children (Brazelton & Greenspan, 2001; Davidson & McEwen, 2012; Vance et al., 2010).

Also, parents who seek mental health treatment communicate to their children that it is crucial to attend to mental health. This display opens up awareness and acceptance that emotional struggles do exist, can be discussed openly, and can be helped. In addition to mental health treatment, such as psychotherapy or medication, parents always benefit from adding social support and self-care to their lives.

As mental health practitioners, it is incumbent upon us to be sensitive to the fact that overly taxed parents benefit far more from encouragement to make small steps to tend to themselves than from judgment for lacking self-care. Also, cultural, historical, economic, and personality factors must be considered in these discussions, as some parents may feel self-care is impossible or contrary to their values. Any way parents can support themselves will benefit the whole family.

10

Treatment Interventions: Transforming the Emotional Climate of the Family

Adults set the tone for the home environment. Children reside in, soak up, and virtually breathe in the emotional climate created by their parents. When families seek therapy, the therapist has an opening to look at and help tune the family's emotional system. To this end, this chapter discusses ways to help children and their parents better understand and express emotions.

If emotions have been avoided or dysregulated in the past, maybe for multiple generations, then parents need help acknowledging their feelings and building their own capacity for emotional regulation before they can help their children recognize and manage their emotions. This work can transform the family environment by focusing not only on the adult's emotional intelligence but also on their parenting practices.

RESPONDING TO CHILDREN'S EMOTIONS

It is crucial, beginning in infancy, for caregivers to respond to children's emotions. Humans are wired to share feelings and to help one another

149

soothe in a crisis. A crying baby is expressing something. Whether or not the parent can solve the problem, attending to the child and making an effort to comfort them is essential. Emotional awareness and coping skills begin within these attachment relationships.

In infancy, parents are almost entirely responsible for comforting their children. Aside from some rudimentary self-soothing skills (thumb sucking, for example), the responsibility for soothing falls on caregivers. They are the ones who help infants recover when they are emotionally upset and introduce them to positive experiences of joy, play, and calm serenity.

The job of parents is to help their children learn to regulate their minds and bodies back to *homeostasis*: balance. This emotional regulation is like a thermostat, moving them away from discomfort and back to a sense of safety and calm. When children are upset, parents take some action to gradually move them from suffering and out of sorts to a state of comfort and ease. As children grow, they can recreate the soothing patterns they learn from their parents. Children often seek out parents when upset or try to copy what parents have done to help them, such as rocking, getting in bed and curling up, or using soothing thoughts and sayings learned from their parents. Over time, children become more and more independent in handling the day-to-day upsets inherent in every life.

Caring, supportive parents reduce the long-term consequences of stress. It only takes one secure adult caregiver to help children buffer stress and aid in coping with adversity. A calm and relaxed adult can guide a child to a state of calm through coregulation. In a safe and attuned relationship, or in times of positive respectful play with an adult, the attachment hormone oxytocin—an antidote to stress—is released. Oxytocin has a relaxing effect on the body and mind and helps in the formation of relational bonding. These relationship qualities, not surprisingly, comprise the 7 essential attachment needs: safety, soothing, attunement, reliability, support, fun, and respectful boundaries.

Children have varying sensitivities to the ups and downs of life and different levels of intensity in their emotional responses to these ups and downs. Awareness of these natural variations in children's responses to stress can help parents better accommodate their needs.

CHILDREN'S DIFFERENT EMOTIONAL TYPES

Emotionally calm children are often quite unruffled. They take life in stride and react in a moderated way to hurt feelings, worries, and things that make them angry. These children often have a wide window of tolerance; they can withstand a lot without getting upset.

A second group of completely normal children is *emotionally intense* and will react with high intensity to the same situations. They may cry disconsolately, tantrum, or panic. While this is occasionally a sign of an emotional disorder, more often this elevated responsiveness is merely a hallmark of a more emotionally intense child. Emotionally intense children are not disordered—they are passionate. They need extra positive attention and a concerted focus on learning to manage their strong feelings and expand their window of tolerance.

Emotionally intense children are often described as intense from birth. Very often, parents will acknowledge their own lifelong emotional intensity and laughingly concur with the notion that the apple doesn't fall far from the tree.

Children with *attachment-related issues* also often have difficulties with emotion regulation. These children struggle less because of their innate temperament than as a result of dysfunctional patterns created in response to very stressful early environments. They have been exposed to high levels of disruption within their primary relationship or have not received support in learning to settle after an emotional upset, and they have not received what they need to develop self-soothing abilities. As a result, they may enter later childhood with weak skills for managing emotions.

Children with early attachment disruptions, separation from the primary caregiver, neglect, or abuse often fall into this category. These children may seem entirely overwhelmed by their own emotions and may seem to overreact to emotional stimulation, flaring dramatically when emotionally aroused. When experiencing strong negative emotions, these children may seem unable to get past them. Such children may get themselves into trouble, often by behaving in ways that are unacceptable to those around them when they are upset: being destructive, hitting, screaming, insulting, running off, or harming themselves. While this type of behavior can have other causes, difficulty tolerating and managing unpleasant feelings is a common root of these types of behavior problems.

Alternatively, some children with attachment-related regulation difficulties may seem emotionally disconnected or unresponsive. They may appear shut down, unable to feel much, or restricted in their expressiveness. When children's feelings are not accepted and welcomed, or where children are not taught to manage them, they may attempt to suppress emotions before becoming aware of them to forestall the uncomfortable helplessness they associate with having a feeling.

The fourth type of child is dealing with a serious *mental health disorder*. This group can overlap with the children who have extreme attachment-based problems. This type of child has an innate mental health disorder such as bipolar disorder, severe mood disorder, or a psychotic disorder. Children of this type have extreme and intense moods that are often independent of their situation. These children may fly into a rage with little or no provoking incident. Their sadness, anxiety, or mania appear to have a life of their own, unrelated to the events in their world and out of proportion to any triggering event. This type of disorder usually comes through genetic inheritance or from early trauma affecting the developing brain. Symptoms can impact the functioning of the family and create a painful cycle.

As a mental health practitioner, you are likely to spend your days with emotionally intense children, children with attachment issues, or children with serious mental health disorders. The first step is to take the necessary time at intake to clarify the root of the emotion-regulation difficulty. A strong developmental history is a necessity, including collecting information on children's early care, any separations from parents or changes in caregivers, moves, deaths, or other experiences that may have impacted the caregivers' emotional stability and capacity for warm presence. We also recommend explicitly inquiring about a family history of mental illness in the immediate and extended family.

TEACHING EMOTION REGULATION ACROSS TYPES

All children need to learn emotion regulation, but the type of help they benefit most from varies depending on children's temperament and mental health (Table 10.1).

Children in the emotionally calm group who are developing typically can usually acquire adequate emotion regulation skills through the good-enough parenting they receive. Parents guide these children by offering emotional support and modeling emotional coping skills. For emotionally calm children, the often intuitive acts of their parents—naming feelings, accepting feelings, expressing their own feelings—are enough. They are naturally resilient and absorb these skills easily through observation and practice. When we meet these children for psychotherapy, it is usually after a stressful event like divorce, a death in the family, or a move, all of which can overtax the coping of any child and motivate diligent parents to seek additional support. Sometimes parents seek help for an ongoing issue like a learning disability. With both stressful events or ongoing problems, traditional child psychotherapy approaches including play therapy, art therapy, age-appropriate talk therapy, and psychoeducation are usually adequate to help the child adjust and return to their stable selves.

Emotionally intense children benefit from more diligent direct teaching of emotion regulation skills. In addition to learning to name and accept emotions as a normal part of life, more intense children need to know exactly what expressions of emotion are off-limits (e.g., hitting, spitting, cursing). More importantly, they need to be told clearly what emotional expressions are acceptable. They benefit from having their positive efforts to self-regulate noticed and articulated back to them with approval. This group of children is particularly responsive to highly positive-toned and very clear parenting styles. Often, the implementation of relationship-based parenting is all this group needs.

When working with emotionally intense children, parents must prioritize their own emotion management. A large portion of the therapeutic work is in helping parents remain calm and firm in the face of defiance, outbursts, and other misbehavior. Parents may need to work through some resentment so that they are able and willing to focus on the child vigorously when they are doing well (Stand 2) and consistently respond with emotional neutrality when misbehavior occurs (Stand 1).

These more intense children may also benefit from psychotherapy, which focuses on the identification of feelings and developing a range of coping skills. Child therapists often address this early in therapy—using feeling faces, articulating the feelings expressed by the child or by the characters in their play, creating art around the topic of feelings, and focusing on emotions in general conversation. Establishing emotional awareness and a robust emotional vocabulary is accomplished by modeling acceptance of feelings that emerge and later building coping skills for self-soothing and appropriate emotional expression.

Resources for this work are included in our reference list at the back of this book. Some particularly useful materials are the *What to Do . . .* series by Dawn Huebner (2005), *What to Do When You're Scared and Worried* by J. Crist (2004), and *The Coping Skills Workbook* and game by Lisa M. Schab and Andy Myer (1996).

The group of children that exhibits severe regulation difficulties related to attachment issues requires more intense, focused, longer-term help in learning emotion regulation. These children have a deficit to make up; their brains developed during a deprived or traumatic early childhood, which encoded within them a pathway of escalation. In order to change these now brain-based deficits, treatment must get in under the children's defensive responses, build the basics of trust, and expand on limited regulatory skills, all in ways that induce hope and do not provoke shame. To this end, these children need a full treatment plan that includes parent coaching, family therapy, individual skill building, and experiential therapy. For these children, successful treatment may also include pharmacologic interventions.

The first step is to decrease the chaos in the home and create a high level of parental emotional regulation, which creates the emotional safety that is a prerequisite for secure attachment to be built (recall the 7 essential attachment needs). For this, we recommend teaching parents a highly structured, clear, and supportive parenting style.

Once the home environment is stabilized, attachment-focused family

Table 10.1 SUMMARY: WAYS TO IMPROVE EMOTION REGULATION ACROSS TEMPERAMENTS AND TYPES	
Temperament and Type	Helpful Interventions
Emotionally Calm	Offer support, guidance, and modeling, traditional psychotherapy, build coping skills, focus on successes in emotion regulation
Emotionally Intense	High levels of recognition for child emotional regulation, consistent modeling of emotion regulation from adults, clear rules for behavior, consistent limit setting for rule breaking, refusal to escalate or debate in response to rule breaking, direct teaching of emotion regulation
Attachment Issues	Very high levels of recognition for emotional regulation, creation of emotional safety by reliable emotion regulation from adults, clear rules for behavior, consistent limit setting for rule breaking, refusal to escalate or debate in response to rule breaking, individual psychotherapy for emotion regulation skill building and processing trauma, attachment-focused family therapy, bottom-up interventions such as biofeedback, occupational therapy, Theraplay
Mental Health disorder	Very high levels of recognition for emotional regulation, clear rules for behavior, consistent limit setting for rule-breaking, refusal to escalate or debate in response to rule breaking, individual psychotherapy for emotion regulation skill building and symptom management skills, possible medication

psychotherapy, individual psychotherapy (play therapy for younger children and relational approaches for older children), and age-appropriate physical interventions such as occupational therapy, meditation, biofeedback, and yoga can be implemented effectively. A particularly useful intervention is Core Attachment Therapy, which is described in detail in *Core Attachment Therapy: Secure Attachment for the Adopted Child* by Dorothy Derapelian (2015).

For children with a more severe mental health disorder, many of the above interventions are useful. While trust and attachment are not the primary focus, families that have been impacted by a severe mental illness can require therapeutic intervention to adjust family patterns. Children who have lived the highly intense and erratic emotional reality of mental illness have often discovered the sad truth that their emotions cannot be regulated through coping skills alone.

These children need stability first, which may require medical intervention. Once stability has been attained, parents and therapists can focus on creating strong structure at home and school, monitoring stress and keeping the tension low, recognizing early signs of relapse, and managing symptoms.

It is also important to work with these children to develop their confidence in regulating themselves emotionally. Normal feelings that other children might take in stride can be difficult for a child with a mental health disorder to tolerate—until she recognizes that there is such a thing as normal sadness, and that it does not always lead to depression. These children also benefit from high-quality, strict, positively toned parenting approaches such as NHA and physiologically based interventions such as yoga and biofeedback.

POSTTRAUMATIC STRESS RECOVERY: A SPECIAL CASE IN MENTAL HEALTH

Posttraumatic stress disorder is a mental health disorder that requires particular attention because a wider variety of interventions may be needed. Children can experience trauma in their families, from neighborhood violence, or from a single-incident trauma such as an automobile accident. The treatment approach will vary depending on whether the traumatic experience is over or ongoing; sadly, we cannot always facilitate the removal of children from traumatizing situations.

Immediate emotional support can make a big difference for children who experience trauma and can minimize trauma's long-term consequences. A safe, caring, and reliable environment is critical to the recovery process. If safety and healing are not available from parents, children are more likely to develop symptoms of depression or anxiety. A secure adult can transfer feelings of safety and calm through coregulation. Predictable, stable, consistent routines also add to feelings of security and have the effect of decreasing children's emotional strain at home.

Both parenting and therapeutic care of traumatized children require a particular mindset: one that recognizes that children are struggling with extreme pain, and that misbehavior is just a sign of that struggle. It is a difficult but powerful process. Holding the calm and boundaried position of setting limits, not taking misconduct personally, and tending first to self-regulation whenever dealing with emotional children is helpful and reduces overall strain. This position puts caregivers in a place of strength and stability rather than reactivity.

Immediate Posttrauma Care

Listed in the box are some powerful interventions to reduce stress and aid in recovery after traumatic events. In the professional literature, there are many sources of insight and clinical interventions for the treatment of trauma and extreme adversity (Baylin & Hughes, 2016; Brunk et al., 1987; Cassidy et al., 2013; Chen et al., 2018; Cohen et al., 2017; Fischer, 2017; Greenberg et al., 1990; Levine, 2015; Ogden et al., 2006; Pennebaker, 2004; Schore, 2001; Shonkoff et al., 2012; van der Kolk, 2015). The box lists the steps we recommend, based on our experience and review of the literature:

EARLY POSTTRAUMATIC INTERVENTION

- Increase overall security
  - Create safety
  - Increase structure
  - Act as attuned, compassionate caregivers
- Reduce overall stress
  - Decrease demands on child temporarily
- Reduce shame, blame, and stigma
  - Normalize biological responses to stress

- Provide psychoeducation for child and parent about trauma reaction
- Don't blame the victim—even when behavior is extreme
- Build on strengths: focus beyond vulnerability
  - Build self-esteem and confidence by pointing out assets and successes
  - Create opportunities for and encourage play and joy
- Attend to body–brain connection
  - Physical activity
  - Teach parent and child relaxation and self-soothing techniques
- Family, friends, and community support
  - Connect with others for fun and warmth
  - Child can choose to talk about past trauma, or not, at their discretion and pace
  - Demonstrate that significant adults can tolerate the truth of the child's trauma
- Parallel treatment for parents
  - Address parental trauma symptoms and emotional reactions to child's trauma
- Individual child psychotherapy
  - Create a trauma narrative (only after above steps are in place, and with researched methods)
  - Challenge self-blaming or nonhelpful thinking

Therapists can start with guiding caregivers to increase security, reduce children's overall stress, and increase positives in the home environment. Such environmental interventions are not insignificant; they provide vital stability to children and are prerequisites for any deeper work. Without safety and stability, the child's nervous system is unable to settle enough to be thoughtful, tolerate painful memories, and learn skills for coping.

To this end, attention can be given to increasing structure and predictability, which is soothing to distressed children. Daily schedules and routines should be created if they have been absent—and adhered to more assiduously than in easy times. Adults supporting a traumatized child should be counseled to be stable and predictable; when children can count on adults to be calm and warm, even in the face of troubles, they can relax more readily. Buffering children from high levels of conflict or instability increases their feelings of security.

In the name of decreasing stress, demands on children can be temporarily lowered. This is not the time to add new responsibilities or push children to take new steps toward independence. Taking a step back in the short term allows them to focus resources on coping and healing. For example, moving a child out of a sibling's bedroom or having him begin walking to school alone in the period immediately following a traumatic event would be ill-timed.

After a traumatic experience, children often regress. They benefit from being allowed to revert to an earlier level of functioning, regroup, and then reestablish their prior level of functioning before being expected to advance. Fun and positive social interactions with caring people aid in healing. Bonding hormones such as oxytocin calm the nervous system and counteract tension. Attention to these environmental components of healing allows children to have the positive experiences needed to feel protected and to see the world as safe and welcoming again.

When parents are coached to focus their attention and enthusiasm on children's successes with minimal attention to current weaknesses or challenges, they help children see themselves in a positive light rather than identifying themselves with negativity or damage associated with a traumatic experience. This building-up effect is especially powerful when provided by both family and therapists.

Caring for Parents of Traumatized Children

Pediatric manifestations of trauma are not just emotional, they are often behavioral. Working with parents to remain calm and regulated—even if a child's behavior is worrisome, annoying, or even infuriating—assists in healing.

The points of care described above require extensive parental involvement and effort. They also require a great deal of parental self-regulation. And all of these demands are placed on parents at a time when they are likely highly stressed, as a trauma experienced by a child usually also takes a huge toll on the child's parents. Parents may struggle with guilt or self-blame around steps they believe they should have taken to protect their child. They may grieve for the child and feel anxious about their child's safety. They may also feel burdened by the pressure of parenting a child who is emotionally and behaviorally dysregulated.

It follows that simultaneous care of the parent of a traumatized child may be necessary. This care may include psychoeducation to normalize the child's and the parents' trauma responses, instilling hope, and building coping skills for managing painful emotions. Any trauma symptoms experienced by the parent will need to be addressed, and the parent will benefit from ongoing support in implementing structure, maintaining regulation in the face of challenges, and nurturing a positive connection with their child.

TRAUMATIZED CHILDREN

Children tend to blame themselves for what happens to them. They lack the maturity to understand that traumatic events are beyond their control; these adverse events in their lives are due to external circumstances. In therapy, psychoeducation and emotion regulation work support children in recognizing that it's normal to have emotional and physical reactions after trauma, that they are not crazy, that they are not being punished, that the trauma was not their fault, and that patience is needed for healing.

Traumatized children can benefit from the type of support that would typically be given to younger children, including more coregulation and heavier reliance on physical interventions, instead of talking interventions. Self-regulation skills can be taught and assigned as homework with parental support, including breathing exercises, physical activity, and calming experiences such as listening to music or bathing. Mindful breathing exercises help to reduce negative tension after trauma and reconnect the trauma survivor with their own body. Physical activity can be emotionally grounding, reducing negative thought cycles and increasing positive energy and feelings of hope. Play helps children recover through reconnection with fun and joy.

Finally, when all else is in place, children may benefit from therapy to directly address the traumatic event. In order to avoid amplifying the trauma, this step should only be added after all prior steps have been addressed. Development of a trauma narrative, work on correcting misconceptions and eliminating self-blame, and utilizing exposure to decrease reactivity are all empirically supported interventions for childhood trauma. For guidelines on using these interventions effectively and ethically, please see our references including Baylin and Hughes (2016) and Cohen et al. (2017).

Top-Down and Bottom-Up Repair

Recovery from trauma is bidirectional: brain to body (top-down) and body to brain (bottom-up). It follows that trauma healing can be approached through the mind or the body (Fosha et al., 2009; van der Kolk, 2015).

Top-down treatment introduces cognitive skills to help reduce distressing and intrusive thoughts, thereby increasing positive, calm feelings in the body. This approach can consist of emotionally supportive talk with adults, learning to use self-soothing words, or cognitive skills training for emotional regulation.

Bottom-up treatment focuses on body awareness and physiological self-soothing: gentle breathing exercises, progressive muscle relaxation, soothing movement, or guided meditation practices. These activities help the child reconnect with their body and mind in positive ways after trauma. Mindful meditation practices, in particular, increase subcortical structures that create a sense of peace and help to manage stress (see recommendations under Mindful and Regulation Tools, later in this chapter).

Research suggests participation in age-appropriate mindfulness activities such as yoga and mindful breathing can significantly reduce PTSD symptoms in children and adolescents (Fischer, 2017; Greenberg & Harris, 2012). Additional physical interventions that have been proven useful are biofeedback, exercise, yoga, tai chi, play therapy, and experiential therapies such as occupational therapy.

We recommend an integrated treatment approach that uses both top-down and bottom-up interventions. Trauma Focused CBT (Cohen et al., 2017), an evidence-based model for the simultaneous treatment of children and their parents, is a powerful intervention that fits this description. It directly addresses the family impact of trauma and has been proven effective for trauma's emotional and behavioral symptoms.

EMOTIONAL FIRST AID: INTERACTING WITH DISTRESSED CHILDREN

Anger and hurt, sadness and jealousy, disappointment and fear are just a few examples of emotions that are no fun to feel. One of the best and kindest things we can do for children is to allow them to feel these emotions in our presence and to be safe and accepted while exploring them. When children's emotions are highly charged—whether due to past trauma or for other reasons—certain approaches can help them cope and regulate overwhelming or very painful feelings.

Allowing children to have, feel, and express their troublesome emotions means not distracting them from pain; not ignoring or playing down the emotions; and not telling them to see the bright side of the situation. Instead, adults can let them notice and experience these unpleasant feelings as they arrive, rise, crest, and fall back. It is in going through this process in a supportive connection that children build the ability to accept and tolerate painful emotions. The most difficult part of this, for parents, is that it can be emotionally excruciating for them to be still and quiet and see their children suffer. But this provision of an accepting and understanding place for tough feelings ultimately honors the emotions and the child.

It is valuable to discuss managing children's emotions with parents. Many times, parents are relieved to hear that they don't need to be a therapist, and that they can connect to their children's feelings in a way that feels right to them as long as their approach includes the following fundamentals.

Recognize the feeling. Name the feeling that is present, or allow children to articulate and name it. Allow children to correct parents if their guess about the feeling is wrong or incomplete. Inquire about the feeling. Listen; simply allow the feeling to exist.

Do not criticize. Avoid belittling or correcting feelings. All emotions are okay for children to have, even if parents are not comfortable with the feeling. Even if parents see the feeling as bratty, irrational, inappropriate, or out of proportion—the emotion belongs to the child, and they get to experience it. This does not mean that every behavioral expression of emotion is okay, however. Help the child to discern the difference between having a feeling and acting it out in harmful ways. Teaching children how to experience and name difficult feelings without being compelled to negatively act them out is good psychotherapy and good parenting.

Do not try to fix it. Help parents learn to tolerate children's discomfort. Parental attitudes of "Let me fix it for you, honey!" preempt children's own coping and communicate intolerance of the emotions or lack of trust that children can tolerate and manage their own feelings. Gentle, attentive presence and warm responsiveness to the child's talk about the feeling or to their physical reaching out may be enough. Of course, after giving children time to manage their emotions and realizing that they cannot, it is useful to intervene and help children calm. This is coregulation.

Avoid overinvolvement. Educate parents on the difference between accepting and assisting versus being taken over by children's emotions (for example, where the parent believes that everything must stop until the child feels better). This occurs most often when parents are swept up in the child's feelings and do not have an adequate emotional boundary with their child. Where parents tend to be overinvolved, their upset may become as intense as the child's—which creates insecurity for the child. Parents who tend to lean in this direction can work on their own emotion management to provide greater security for their children in moments of upset.

Moving on. It can be tricky to distinguish feelings that need expression from those that children are getting stuck in and having trouble moving beyond. There is a sweet spot in honoring, but it dissipates when we get lost in feelings. Therapists know and parents can learn to intuit that point where further discussion is not helpful and it is time to transition to something physical or distracting. Being a responsive parent does not mean dwelling on every feeling every time. It is also important to not accidentally teach children that being upset is their most reliable path to receiving attention and intimacy; parents should take care to demonstrate often that attention is also available in moments of happiness and success.

Overreactions. If children appear to be overreacting, parents can respond with curiosity. Why are they overreacting now? Are they tired? Hungry? Sick? Did they have a problem at school that has left them feeling bad? These would be feelings to acknowledge. Teach parents to be wary of their own anger or fear response when their child overreacts; when they are triggered, they may escalate the interaction unnecessarily.

Safety. If safety is at risk, of course, parents must intervene to protect the child and others—physically, if necessary. However, even in these rare circumstances, it is not helpful to ignore, criticize, attempt to eradicate, overindulge, or react with high levels of emotionality to children's feelings. As soon as safety is reestablished, parents can go back to the other fundamentals described above.

As parents develop attachment-sound practices, therapists should be clear that while compassion for children's feelings is necessary, they do not need to alter their decisions or forestall limit setting in response to those feelings. Recognizing children's emotions does not mean that they will be able to have their wishes met. It is entirely possible and even helpful to say to children, "I see you are angry, but we are not going to the park" or "You are feeling very sad because playtime is over." Notice that setting a limit does not require disconnection or ignoring children's feelings; they can coexist.

Parents can't overnurture children, but they can overprotect children. Protecting children from the discomfort of their negative emotions can undermine their learning to manage those feelings. Most difficult emotions children experience are painful, but not damaging or devastating. It is critical to distinguish between helping and interfering in children's natural emotional processes. While painful feelings are distressing for parents to witness, their ability to sit with their discomfort and accept seeing their children in pain communicates that emotions are natural, tolerable, a part of life, and not an emergency. These are important topics for discussion with parents.

Keep in mind that children do not only need negative emotions to be recognized by adults; they also need their positive emotions to be embraced.

Parent–child play, laughter, and surprise are all essential to building connections with children and guiding them toward knowing and feeling comfortable with all their emotions. Helping children regard their joyful moments helps them develop their identities as people capable of joy, whose lives include great pleasure. It is also fun for parents. Attending primarily to painful feelings and not responding equally to happiness can create a lopsided self-view that focuses on negative emotions.

Therapist Note: A Sensitive Balance

Therapists are also not immune to the desire to protect children from painful emotions. In working with children, watch your comfort with different emotions. Note whether you are shifting the focus when children are expressing pain. Perhaps you catch yourself jumping to problem solving rather than allowing the feelings to exist or engaging in other subtle ways of moving away from children's painful feelings.

On the other hand: Never press children to stay with painful feelings beyond their willingness and interest. Excessive focus on negative emotions can inadvertently create an identity around being damaged. It can cause the child to develop a dislike for therapy or to make a habit of amplifying misery. Be sure also to encourage fun and play in your therapy office!

To assist parents in developing comfort with emotions, actively ask about their responses to their children's pleasant and unpleasant feelings, their own comfort with different feelings, what feelings and behaviors trigger them, and their emotional self-care. Engage parents in a discussion of their own emotions when setting limits with children, and how they can set boundaries without disconnecting. Also, encourage them to discuss their feelings about reconnection after conflicts.

TEACHING CHILDREN TO UNDERSTAND FEELINGS

A central task of family therapists (and parents) is to familiarize children with their emotional lives, validate their feelings, and help in the development of emotion regulation skills. Emotion regulation is not about suppressing feelings, or just venting feelings; it is about learning to recognize them, accept them, and utilize them for decision making, agency, and boundary setting.

Children and adults often attribute their feelings solely to the actions of others rather than to their own personal, internal processes. It is typical for children to say and believe, if they feel angry at someone's behavior, "He made me mad." When they are anxious about a perceived slight, a child will say, "She made me upset." Many children can engage in discussion around the idea that emotions do not come directly from external sources; they come from inside of people and provide them with information about themselves and what they like or dislike about situations. It is important to discuss with children (and parents too!) that no one can make them feel a certain way. Feelings are information that they generate within themselves based on their temperament, history, and interpretation of the current situation.

This insight about emotions as an internal process is powerful and can be challenging for some to grasp, particularly for children. It is worth working to develop this perspective, however, because it gives children power and puts emotional control back into their hands. Once children understand that their feelings belong to them, they can take steps to use them to communicate, set limits, or change what they are doing or thinking. Like adults, children can learn to shift their dialogue to "I feel mad" or "I notice I'm feeling upset." With guidance, modeling, and practice, children can learn to appropriately express their feelings and to use self-talk to put feelings into perspective. They can learn to say, "He was rude, but I can ignore him," or "There are no cookies, but I can have some ice cream."

PARENTS AS ROLE MODELS FOR EMOTION

Parents can best support a child's development of emotional awareness and regulation when they are proficient at understanding and regulating their own feelings. This process is particularly challenging and important when emotions are heated. There are at least three good reasons for parents to self-regulate when a child is acting out or misbehaving:

1. Escalating or flaring in frustration at one's children has a negative impact on those children's ability to emotionally regulate. When parents yell or even scold children, it heats up the interaction rather than calming it. Most children respond to parental escalation with heightened agitation and emotionality.

2. Flaring parents are role models for escalation, which suggests to children that these behaviors are acceptable expressions of anger.

3. Some children find passionate parental responses alluring. This is a basic tenet of NHA: Some children feel compelled to repeat actions that turn on their parents' intensity. This does not mean that these children like being yelled at; it is the passion of the response that hooks them. Consider roller coasters: If you like them, would you say they are enjoyable? Most people say that they are not exactly pleasant, but that they are exciting and stimulating. The reaction of some emotionally intense children to parental outbursts reflects the same kind of experience of adult emotionality. Additionally, most children love being the center of attention—especially of a parent's attention—and parents typically shift to high levels of focus and responsiveness when negative behaviors or negative feelings are in the mix. This can inadvertently communicate to children that they are more valued or interesting when they are misbehaving or suffering. This imbalance can create in children a pattern of seeking intimacy and connection principally through acting out or suffering and seeking support, rather than in a healthier pattern of knowing adults are there when they are unhappy but that they are equally available for positive experiences. (Therapists take note: We can also be guilty of this.)

For parents to maintain a consistently unflappable, steady, trustworthy, helpful state, it is useful for them to build a practice around emotional recovery. They can build a habit of noticing when they start to tense up, escalate, lecture, or criticize, and to take these moments as cues to return to a calm state before engaging children. Parents can take a deep breath, walk away, consciously disconnect from conflict, and reengage with peaceful parts of themselves. This practice not only serves to calm parents but also calms their children by slowing and calming the interaction.

Parents often find it quite challenging to self-calm in the heat of conflict; they feel pressure to make children's misbehavior stop, to end the annoyance, or to otherwise get them to do what the parents want. In this frame of mind, it is natural to feel resistance to self-monitoring and self-soothing, as the children's behavior feels like the priority. Changing focus to regulating one's own tension is difficult, but parents and children benefit when they can acknowledge that the real priority is parent self-regulation. Soothe and regulate first; then, turn to problems.

Self-Reset for Emotion Regulation

Therapists and parents can use the concept of resetting to help themselves recover emotionally. Resetting is part of the work of parenting. When we reset ourselves, we do a 180-degree about-face from a position of tension, pressure, and impulsivity to a position of calm and thoughtfulness. Self-reset is accomplished by prioritizing calm over emotional reactivity and being willing to take whatever time is necessary to settle oneself. Sometimes a reset can be performed in seconds; other times, it takes much longer.

In resetting themselves, parents de-energize conflict. A self-reset expresses that whatever is transpiring is not the way to get the parent to react animatedly or otherwise lean in. The nonverbal message is: "I do not escalate when things are going wrong; I am not activated by misbehavior." Resetting one's self is a vital part of Stand 1 (Absolutely No); the use of resets as consequences is part of Stand 3 (Absolutely Clear). Stand 3 resets are covered in much more detail later in Part IV.

The real benefit of parents learning to reset themselves is role modeling. Children who see their parents intentionally reset will learn to imitate this skill.

Fostering Emotion Regulation

Parents tend to spend a lot of time scolding children for mismanaging their emotions. While the parents' intentions in bringing focus to the failing are usually good—an effort to make their children aware that their way of acting out an emotion is a problem, and to support them in making a better effort in the future—this method often fails.

Scolding actually results in children feeling angry, hurt, or misunderstood, and can create a sense of "Why bother? I can't do this right." Therapists can guide parents away from pointing out failures in children's emotion regulation and toward focusing attention on moments of successful regulation. Pointing out successes to children strengthens confidence and willingness to keep trying. It enhances their awareness that success is possible.

Stand 2 can be employed as an impactful intervention for teaching children to express feelings appropriately. Parents can practice recognizing children for any aspect of emotion recognition or management, even if it is small. Intentionally engaging in this practice of recognition is a way of increasing the parents' attention to, and enthusiastic response to, any behavior their children exhibit that is excellent, good, okay, or even not as bad as usual, which in turn increases the child's awareness of their own success.

REVIEW OF THE 3 STANDS

The core principles of NHA:

Stand 1: Absolutely No—Adults do not react passionately to children's negativity, mistakes, or misbehavior. They do not allow negativity to be a focal point of the adult-child relationship.

Stand 2: Absolutely Yes—Adults relentlessly seek out and focus on children's positivity and success. They appreciate, acknowledge and nurture experiences of success, no matter how small.

Stand 3: Absolutely Clear—Adults are clear about rules and expectations and hold these in a steady way. Adults set no limit with harshness, nor emphasize failure in any way.

To focus on fostering emotion regulation, therapists can teach parents to comment in a detailed, enthusiastic way on children's efforts to express or manage their feelings. For example, "I see you used good judgment in walking away when your sister yelled at you. I can see from your face you are upset, but you stayed calm, asked her to stop, and then left when she did not stop. You are showing good self-control." Or "Even though you dislike broccoli, I notice that you did not complain. You left it on your plate and just focused on eating your chicken. You were successful in avoiding whining and fussing." In each of these cases, parents are highlighting to children their in-the-moment success in noticing and managing feelings. Notice the detailed, positive descriptions of the children's reactions.

Children often fail to notice what they did well; feedback like this supports them in beginning to recognize the small steps they are already taking toward handling their feelings better. When parents describe children's incontrovertible successes to them, children can take this in and feel proud. Typically, this kind of feedback inspires children to redouble their efforts to continue those behaviors.

MINDFUL PARENTING: DEALING WITH NEGATIVITY

Children are not always gratifying, nor should they be. Parenting is much easier in good times. In the rough and tumble of daily life, parents can be especially challenged by children's negative feelings, or by behavior that provokes negativity in the parents. For example, when children hurt their parents' feelings or offend them, the parents might react aggressively or withdraw, or might yield to the children's demands to avoid further upset.

During these moments, parents can be encouraged to remain calm and aware of their own emotions, while compassionately noticing their children's emotions—a form of mindful awareness.

Mindful parenting aligns with the qualities that form a secure attachment, including paying attention, offering attunement, and creating safety. Mindfulness also plays a preventative role—practicing mindfulness can allow parents to be more resistant to negative feelings and feel more positive feelings in stressful situations (Farb et al., 2014).

Holding a mindful stance is easiest when life is calm and going well; however, it is most important when life is not peaceful and things are difficult.

If parents can develop the ability to be steady in tough moments, they can share that composure with their children rather than joining in children's chaos. This positive dynamic avoids high stress, escalation, and later remorse for both parents and children, and it models and teaches self-regulation to children. Parents cultivating a mindfulness practice regularly—between crises—train their nervous systems to more readily default to a mindful state when things feel chaotic. In addition, mindfulness is a critical component of employing relationship-based parenting. Following the 3 Stands requires that parents hold clear intentions, self-regulate, be patient, and attune in the moment.

When children are more demanding, or caregivers are tired, frustrated, or upset, it is easy to fall off the mindful path. It is normal, tempting, and very human to be swept up by interactions that seem problematic and to allow this magnetic draw toward problems to dominate the response and subsequent parent–child interactions. Where parents' stress is chronically high, or where their own upbringing was marked by trauma or attachment problems, the threshold for shifting into fight-or-flight mode and overreacting to negative stimuli is lowered. While this is understandable, it is less productive than maintaining a positive or neutral stance.

Parents benefit from practicing reset in therapy sessions and at home by shifting conscious attention to their breathing and bodily sensations. Have them notice: Are they breathing quickly or slowly? Are they feeling calm, tense, or tired? What thoughts are running through their minds? Building awareness of their own thoughts and feelings in the moment can help them regulate themselves and better observe the needs of their children.

As parents learn to reset and feel into the experience of a more mindful state, therapists can guide them to notice that this state allows them to pay closer attention to their children in the moment—an essential component of creating security. Ask parents to apply their new mindfulness skills to observing the overall intensity and timing of children's nonverbal cues, including eye contact, facial expressions, tone of voice, posture, gestures, and touch. Dan Siegel (2015) describes in his book, *Brainstorm,* the power of this kind of observation in parental support of the development of children's inner emotional lives.

MINDFULNESS FOR PARENTS

As therapists, we recognize that in the context of busy daily life, it's easy to lose track of parenting intentions. Introducing mindful reflection into their lives requires a commitment of time, which can be particularly difficult for pressured parents. However, even a short mindful activity, when practiced with regularity, can improve parents' peace of mind and calm family interactions. We are not suggesting that it is easy for parents to establish a regular mindfulness practice. Even skilled meditation practitioners find it takes a conscious effort every week, every day, and sometimes every minute to return to thoughtful attention.

One popular mindfulness approach is the mindfulness-based stress reduction program developed by Jon Kabat-Zinn, MD, which combines self-awareness exercises, cognitive coping skills, movement, and simple meditation options for calming the mind. These classes can offer parents and therapists a place to nurture themselves and find resilience in their interactions with children. Research has found that these programs have emotional and physical benefits such as improved emotional awareness, reduced fear responses, a strengthened immune system, and pain reduction (Kabat-Zinn, 1982; Kabat-Zinn et al., 1992; Lazar, 2016). Mindful meditation can help with emotional distress by reducing negative thoughts and raising self-compassion (Farb et al., 2014; Williams et al., 2007).

Example: Mindfulness Breathing Exercise

Here is a simple guided mindfulness exercise you can share with parents who are just beginning to explore mindfulness:

> Take a moment to slow your breath and let your body get comfortable where you are sitting. Focus on your breathing, in and out, without overfocusing on any thoughts that pop into your mind. Let thoughts float by like clouds. Repeatedly bring yourself back to this moment by paying attention to your breath.
>
> Now, take five slow, deep breaths in and out. If your mind gets

distracted, that is okay; remind yourself just to breathe. Breathing in, tell yourself, "I am breathing in." Breathing out, tell yourself, "I am breathing out." Feel the movement in your chest and abdomen as you breathe. Let your body relax.

Notice what you feel when you slow down, even for less than a minute. Your nervous system can start to relax. This is the beginning of the practice of mindful meditation.

MINDFULNESS FOR CHILDREN

Research also strongly supports the use of age-appropriate mindfulness practices with children and adolescents. Breathing exercises, progressive muscle relaxation, guided meditation, yoga, and tai chi have shown promise with this population. Evidence suggests that mindfulness skills can improve children's emotional regulation, concentration, memory, and learning (Burke, 2010; Coatsworth et al., 2009; Harrison et al., 2004; McGreevy, 2011; van de Weijer-Bergsma et al., 2012).

Traditional psychotherapy techniques such as teaching children to acknowledge, identify, and manage emotions are based on mindfulness. They improve mood, create resilience, and build confidence. Even cognitive-behavioral therapy practices, such as stopping negative thought cycles, are achieved through mindful awareness and self-regulation.

Mindful practices tend to be self-reinforcing, since they promote feelings of peace and reduce negativity. The sense of calm and positivity they generate increases the likelihood that children will use the skills again in the future. If children do not learn the skills needed to cope with negative thoughts or moods, they can easily get caught in negative cycles of worry and self-criticism. However, over time, mindfulness skills can serve to reduce these distorted thoughts and feelings of anxiety, which can then foster development of long-term patterns of positivity rather than negativity (Burns, 2008; Farb et al., 2014).

Although these skills can be self-reinforcing, children still benefit from parents pointing out their successes with mindfulness tools and commenting appreciatively on their improved emotional resilience. As we have been discussing, children—and humans in general—tend to have difficulty noting small, incremental improvements. Children benefit from having such improvements pointed out to them in clear, undeniable ways.

As part of a family psychotherapy approach, providers can teach parents to model mindful coping skills themselves at home. We recommend parents announce out loud and publicly their plan to take some breaths, take a break, or go for a walk with the goal of calming, and then do so. This process helps children consciously learn self-calming skills through observation and gives them a chance to witness their parents avoiding an emotional meltdown or harsh response to them. Parents can also help children with mindful activities through direct teaching. With practice, self-regulation skills can then become part of children's repertoire for managing intense feelings and reducing problematic behaviors.

Mindfulness and Regulation Tools

The next step for therapists is to teach children specific mindful self-regulation tools. Calming practices of conscious breathing and muscle relaxation can help children with self-soothing and emotional regulation. Even very young children can learn and use these simple relaxation techniques. As children grow in sophistication, their toolbox of skills can grow too. Here are some easy activities to teach and use with children.

Blow out your candle. For this activity, which is ideal for very young children, the adult and child each hold up an index finger like a candle. They then take a deep breath and slowly let it out, as if blowing out a candle. The goal is to exhale entirely, as if the candle were hard to blow out. You can inspire them by telling them this is a chance to practice blowing out however many candles they'll have on their cake at their next birthday.

Blowing soap bubbles. This fun activity can be used to help younger children tune into their breathing, learn to extend it, and experience taking deep breaths. The adult can demonstrate and coach the child in making bigger bubbles by gently and slowly exhaling.

Belly breathing. Have the child lie on their back on the floor or couch. Have them place a small ball on their belly and try to take a breath so deep it causes the ball to roll off. This game is an excellent remedy for children who heave their shoulders while breathing and keep their breath confined to the upper chest. It gives a firsthand example of what it feels like to breathe deeply. Over time, children can transfer this knowledge into breathing more fully while sitting and standing.

Hand on chest and belly breathing. For adolescents, deep breathing can be taught by placing one hand on the chest and one on the lower abdomen. Ask teens to feel the warmth of their hands on their body, focus on their breathing, slow and deepen their breath, and concentrate on their inhale and exhale. Emphasize the importance of exhaling fully, which creates a calming physiological response.

Sound of a bell. Focusing attention on the sound of a bell, listening until you can no longer hear the ring, is a meditative activity. It focuses the mind on the sound at the moment.

Progressive muscle relaxation. To guide children in gradually relaxing their bodies, one muscle group at a time, walk the child through the following steps:

- Have the child lie down and begin taking slow, deep breaths.
- After several deep breaths, tell the child, in a calm and soothing tone, "Bring your attention to your feet. Relax your toes, feet, and ankles."
- Wait briefly, then add, "Now, relax your calves and knees."
- Move slowly up the body regions, one by one, prompting the child to relax thighs, lower back, mid-upper back, belly, chest, shoulders, arms, hands, neck, throat, jaw, mouth, face, eyes, and forehead. Keep in mind that this exercise can also be done from head to toes (top-down) rather than toes to head (bottom-up).

Tension and release. This exercise is similar to the progressive relaxation above, but it involves tightly squeezing a muscle group, then releasing and relaxing it. Holding a muscle group in maximum tension for 5–10 seconds can help the muscles to relax once you release them. For some people—especially those who hold a lot of baseline tension—this is easier than just trying to relax:

- Begin by having the child sit or lie down comfortably.
- Then ask the child to take a deep breath, then exhale; and then to take another deep breath and tense their hands, holding the tension tighter, tighter, for 5–10 seconds. (When they tense the muscles of their hands, make sure they are clear that they are not to tense the arms, shoulders, or any other body part besides the one you named. It might initially be difficult for a child to isolate muscle groups.)
- Next, have the child exhale completely and totally release the tension. The child may notice how different this feels: perhaps warm, or loose, maybe soft.
- Have the child remain in this relaxed state for 10–15 seconds.
- Repeat, moving through the muscle groups: arms, shoulders, neck, face, chest, belly, back, legs, and toes. One by one, instruct the child to tense each muscle group, then relax it.

Once skills are in place, parents can guide these relaxation techniques at home. Children often enjoy the uninterrupted one-on-one attention inherent in these activities. They can be beneficial as a bedtime activity. The children's book *A Boy and a Bear* (Lite, 1996) is a good resource for parents who would like more guidance on deep breathing exercises for young children. In all of these cases, it is important for the adult also to use and demonstrate the skill. Children and teens are more open to an activity that they observe the adult is also willing to practice.

MINDFULNESS FOR TEENS

Emotions are dominant in the teen's experience and tend to be primary drivers for their decision-making processes. It is an exciting and risky time. The teen's brain is wired in ways that push them to separate from family and become increasingly independent. In combination, the drive for independence and the high emotionality typical of the teen years often create strife at home. This is not an easy time for parents to navigate.

A mindful parenting approach can be particularly useful during adolescence. Reflective habits can be great tools to support the push and pull that parents may feel from their teens or within themselves during this phase of quick changes and shifting priorities. When parents practice emotional coping skills, they teach their adolescents to do the same, both directly and indirectly.

For teens, mindfulness activities such as yoga, tai chi, or martial arts can help them cope with the inevitable stresses of change and maturation and to build self-confidence. Over time, mindfulness skills can be integrated into their growing neurological structure and carry through into adulthood. Although brains are flexible throughout the life span, adolescence is a critical time for learning and growing. The brain is actively remaking itself, laying new neurological pathways and pruning those that aren't used (Lester & Sparrow, 2010; Schore, 2015).

MINDFULNESS IN SCHOOLS

> Stress is the number one enemy of public education, especially in inner-city schools. It creates tension and violence and compromises the cognitive and psychological capacity of the student.
>
> JAMES DIERKE,
> A NATIONAL MIDDLE SCHOOL PRINCIPAL OF THE YEAR

> Isn't it ironic that we teach students about everything except themselves?
>
> CARLOS GARCIA,
> PAST SUPERINTENDENT OF SAN FRANCISCO SCHOOLS

Recently, school programs have focused more resources on enhancing emotional and social development, including the addition of mindfulness practices for students and teachers (Burke, 2010; Cassani, 2015; Rothenberg Gritz, 2015). Programs bringing meditation and yoga practices into schools have been found to reduce stress and conflict for children and teachers.

No young child should be expected to meditate like an adult. Even adults struggle to quietly meditate without some guidance. More active and fun adult-guided interventions including body movement and breathing practices are likely to be successful with primary school and middle school children—and with more energetic children of all ages (children that need the most help to calm themselves are likely to find it hard to sit still to meditate).

The following are two examples of successful school-based mindfulness programs.

Mindful Moments Rooms

In Baltimore, Maryland, mindfulness programs were created to reduce stress and trauma for children raised in areas with high rates of violent crime and unemployment. The schools created Mindful Moments Rooms with yoga and meditation for students and teachers to help them cope with anger or other negative emotions. They found the program reduced suspensions to zero. It also offered students an alternative to fighting to cope with stress and conflict. There are now more than a dozen programs in Baltimore, with similar programs in more than 15 states across the country (Sreenivasan, 2017).

Quiet Time

In San Francisco, a meditation program for children called Quiet Time, where children are given time to be quiet and taught to reflect, has been implemented in some schools. The goal is to teach and practice skills to reduce stress reactions at school and at home. A variety of gains have been found to result from this program. Students' academic performance improved and so did their social interactions. They noted less conflict. Another unexpected result was that it also increased teacher retention (Cassani, 2015; David Lynch Foundation, n.d.; Rothenberg Gritz, 2015).

MINDFUL THERAPISTS AND REGULATION IN CHILD PSYCHOTHERAPY

Providers will find it easier to teach mindfulness when they have a routine of their own. Having the personal experience to draw from helps when discussing the value of reflective practice, and it helps the provider model mindfulness in the session. Mindfulness practice helps therapists maintain calm, flexibility, and presence under stress. It also fosters attunement and compassion in their work, both explicitly and implicitly.

Although mindful techniques can be taught, teaching the value of acceptance and patience is most beneficial when modeled in person. We encourage all providers to experiment with a form of reflective practice that fits with their lifestyle. The options are limitless, so let your imagination play.

As a pediatric psychotherapist, it is your job to be present with your patient's dysregulation: to see it and hold the space without being drawn into it or insisting on jumping out of it. It is your primary job to remain connected and observant and to bring regulated, compassionate presence to each moment. This way of being is therapeutic in its own right, and a prerequisite to more targeted, strategic interventions for fostering emotion regulation.

Within this relationship, there is room for many styles of child psychotherapy. Play therapy, cognitive–behavioral work, skill building, art therapy, and talk therapy are all potentially useful. Your choice should depend on your training, the age of the child, and the child's specific needs. In general, we suggest being prepared to work on recognizing, accepting, and expressing feelings, both nonverbally and verbally.

Recognizing. The children brought to see us sometimes have very limited emotional vocabulary and benefit from exposure to the rich vocabulary available to us to describe feelings. Experiences such as creating a continuum of feelings from *bothered* to *enraged* with a list of gradually escalating feeling words can be useful for building emotional vocabulary. Commonly used therapy toys such as feeling faces can be used creatively to open up conversations about feelings. Labeling feelings that show up in conversation or in play, having children create art representing differing feelings, or presenting puppets or toys that are experiencing specific feelings are all ways to normalize and build recognition of a wide array of emotional states.

Accepting. Standard child psychotherapy approaches are very useful in communicating the acceptability of all feelings. With younger children, model acceptance of feelings expressed in art or in play; with older children, normalize feelings revealed in discussion. It is important for child therapists to create a high level of clarity regarding acceptance of feelings and their expression while setting limits on aggression or other kinds of destructive acting out of the feeling. Inform children of office rules—"No hitting; no hurting; no breaking the office"—to put parameters on behavior rather than on feelings.

Expressing. Children are not always able to verbally discuss their experiences and feelings. Good-quality child psychotherapy allows clients to release their feelings both nonverbally and verbally. For nonverbal sharing, child therapist offices should be well supplied with items for drawing and toys for play therapy that encourage full expression of feelings—including aggression and nurturing. Keep in mind that your body language, tone of voice, and facial expression nonverbally convey your awareness of and sympathy for the child's emotional state.

Verbally, it is helpful to notice and articulate your patient's emotions as well as your own when appropriate. Use items such as feeling faces to support a discussion of emotions and to teach techniques children can use to handle difficult feelings overtly. See Lite (1996), Crist (2004), Huebner (2005), and others in the references for useful resources about working with children on emotion regulation.

CONCLUSION: EMOTIONAL AWARENESS AND REGULATION

Emotional awareness and regulation are keystones to the development of a balanced and satisfying life. Like adults, children have naturally varying levels of emotionality. Some are spirited, others more subdued. A central feature of our work as family therapists is to help children and parents accept and enjoy whatever natural level of intensity is present in family members while supporting them in building self-regulation skills.

Not all emotional intensity is natural or healthy. It can be the product of trauma, chronic stress, or mental illness. Even when psychotherapy or medication are needed to bring a child's intensity within healthy bounds, we propose prioritizing parental self-regulation—which equips them to act as role models for their children and to positively influence the emotional tone of the family. Also, gains in parental self-awareness and self-control make it easier for children to feel their emotions and regulate. And finally, regulated parents create a secure home where children's inevitable emotionality can be met with equanimity and safety.

For family therapists, a primary goal in working with parents is to increase their mindful awareness of emotions, both for themselves and for their children. As parents develop skills for mindful parenting, they are better able to do the work required to improve coregulation, teach children self-calming techniques, and build relationship-based parenting practices.

This emotional work happens in synchrony with the building of the parent–child attachment relationship. Attachment and regulation are not independent factors; they are mutually influential. Each one builds on the other, and both are essential for healthy child development. This leads into Part IV, which focuses on emotionally sensitive and attachment-sound learning and discipline.

PART IV

TRANSFORMING BEHAVIOR AND DISCIPLINE

When you plant lettuce, if it does not grow well, you don't blame the lettuce. You look for reasons it is not doing well. It may need fertilizer, or more water, or less sun. You never blame the lettuce. Yet if we have problems with our friends or family, we blame the other person. But if we know how to take care of them, they will grow well, like the lettuce. Blaming has no positive effect at all; nor does trying to persuade using reason and argument. That is my experience. No blame, no reasoning, no argument, just understanding. If you understand, and you show that you understand, you can love, and the situation will change.

THICH NHAT HANH, *AT HOME IN THE WORLD*

11

Orientation to Theory and Science: Relationship-Based Discipline

Previous chapters have laid the foundation for understanding the parent–child relationship from a neurobiological and attachment perspective, as well as strengthening skills for emotional regulation in the family. With these in place, the stage is set to focus on limit setting.

Discipline is daunting for many parents. Caring parents struggle to find the sweet spot for behavior management, wanting to effectively set limits without harming their children. In this part, we focus exactly on this dilemma, laying out attachment-sound and neurobiologically compatible ways to set clear limits with children. Key to this approach is the insight that the best discipline occurs in relational connection and does not require harshness or rupture of the relational flow.

Parents can be highly motivated for this work and often approach therapists with a goal of improved behavior management in mind. For therapists, it can be very rewarding to see positive changes in parents' approaches to discipline—and to watch these changes create improved boundaries in the family, support the personal growth of the child, and decrease parental stress.

Ultimately, the parent–child relationship itself is improved when discipline is managed in a consistent, balanced, regulated manner. Expertise in helping parents with discipline can be a powerful area of competence for therapists.

WHO IS THE CLIENT?

Discipline issues are a common reason that parents seek psychotherapy for their children or parenting support for themselves. And it is common for parents to assume children need individual therapy when behavioral issues are the presenting concern. However, we would recommend that therapists initially shift parental expectations away from child therapy and toward refining parents' skills for dealing with behavior within the power of the parent–child relationship. Many children do not need a therapist working with them to make behavioral changes; parents, given the proper techniques, can affect these changes themselves.

Parents may not realize that without their informed involvement, changes in children's behavior and mood are difficult, if not impossible. The goal is parents becoming therapeutic agents. This is why we suggest that therapy begin with intensive parent training. After this is accomplished, individual treatment for children can be added if still needed.

In our practices, we have found that 60–70% of cases opened for children with emotional outbursts, defiance, or conduct problems can be satisfactorily resolved using parenting training as the primary intervention. For children with more internalized emotional disturbances, front-loading parenting work is also beneficial, although many of these children may still require individual therapy later on.

ADDRESSING DISCIPLINE WITH PARENTS: INITIAL CHALLENGES

The topic of discipline raises powerful feelings in most people. Parents often feel confused by mixed messages from their own past experiences, advice from friends, family expectations, and cultural values. Reputable professionals contradict one another: Some advise greater strictness, while others advocate for more relaxed parenting; some recommend higher levels of engagement and others, more hands-off approaches.

For a parent seeking guidance, the available information can be confusing and overwhelming—particularly when children are more intense or challenging. Parents of these children are likely to have received a lot of feedback that they are at fault for their children's issues. This is not our perspective. While we advise parenting intervention as a first-line approach, it is not because discipline issues are the parents' fault, but rather because parents need more potent and effective methods for their children. It is not the parents that are at fault when children's intensity gets out of hand; it is the techniques at their disposal.

Of course, some parents have limitations in their self-control, insight, or capacity to attune. Even parents with these limitations gain advantages by learning more useful tools. We hold that a neurobiologically based, attachment-sound parenting approach can be taught; and we accept that parents will learn this approach differently, depending on their current level of emotional proficiency. Even the most challenged parents can begin using these skills primarily at a simple behavioral level. With practice and personal growth, they can continue refining their approach, to be ever more accurately attuned to their children, gradually adding greater depth, sensitivity, and attunement.

If parents' own childhoods were filled with primarily healthy parenting experiences, repeating these positive patterns is natural and rewarding. However, if parents' past experiences were mostly negative, they may feel dismayed to observe themselves unconsciously replaying these old antagonistic patterns. To make positive changes in parenting, some caregivers only need psychoeducation and new perspectives. Others require more in-depth interventions, including parent training and individual therapy that patiently allows them the time and support needed to heal and grow. Making parenting intervention an early part of the treatment plan creates an immediately more sound and secure disciplinary environment for children, allowing for more notable psychological changes evolving in parents over time. The effectiveness of family therapists is enhanced by building skills to work at all of these gradations of family needs.

When parents are frustrated because of discipline problems, providers have a unique opportunity to assist them. Addressing these issues is often a sensitive subject for parents, who may feel ashamed or out of control. They may be afraid of negative judgment from the therapist and may seek both emotional reassurance and parenting guidance. Usually, these parents are looking for tools to manage children's behavior and family conflict, but are also open to making more significant changes in family patterns. In this time window, therapists can use their unique skill sets to look at family dynamics and to teach parents strategies to help create productive transformations in families' lives.

Once parents feel that the therapy is safe and secure, they can look at themselves openly and honestly. It can allow a space for parents to reflect on their intentions and what matters in their families. Once they feel safe, learning and change can occur. Here, the parents can develop an approach that is responsive rather than reactive. Instead of allowing children's negative behavior to negatively shift parents' mindsets, parents can focus on regulating themselves to provide stability, consistency, and positivity.

WHY DISCIPLINE MATTERS

Discipline means teaching. When parents are successful in teaching children, the lessons are internalized within children's minds and develop into self-discipline that stays with them for the rest of their lives. Children need to learn self-control to pace themselves in complex situations, to know when to slow down or stop and when to activate or go; parents can learn to both model and teach this kind of self-control.

This modulation is mirrored within the structure of the human autonomic nervous system (ANS). As presented earlier, the ANS has two divisions, the parasympathetic system (PNS)—rest and digest—and the sympathetic system (SNS)—fight or flight. In ordinary times of low to moderate stress, the PNS is dominant, and the individual feels safe and secure enough for the body to relax. In this state, a person can feel calm and social. On the other hand, when the mind perceives urgency or danger, the SNS is dominant, causing the person to feel activated or anxious. In a life-threatening emergency, the crisis portion of the PNS (dorsal vagal) can trigger physical immobilization (collapse) to protect one's life.

Parents' style of discipline interacts directly with their children's nervous systems. When parents are feeling urgency or pushing children to do something, the children are likely to move into a sympathetic state of activation. This approach increases children's feelings of tension and decreases their social engagement. When parents are feeling calm and interacting patiently, children are likely to move into a parasympathetic state of ease. This steady parental stance increases children's feelings of safety and connection. The parent's approach either agitates and shuts down the child's system or relaxes and opens up their bodies and minds to learning.

Children's interactions with reliable and secure parents form a foundation for their immature nervous systems to develop flexibility across different emotional states and life circumstances. This process establishes children's capacity to return to calm stability after stressful events and to interact more easily with the world across various situations. After years of repetition, children gradually learn when and how to activate themselves and when and how to calm down. Fostering this development is a core goal of discipline, teaching, and therapy.

DISCIPLINE MEANS TEACHING

One of the primary jobs of parents is to raise children who are functional, independent, contributing members of society—who can enjoy their relationships and experiences, and then raise the next generation of healthy humans. To this end, parents are working for the future of their children and the world. These lofty parent goals are rarely in mind when a child is misbehaving, annoying others, or being difficult. The natural urge of parents at that moment is to make it stop. But discipline is for the future, not for the present moment.

Discipline and teaching are inseparable. Children are sponges, continuously learning even when parents do not think they are learning things. How parents implement discipline will influence what lessons their children take away. Will they learn what the parent is trying to teach, or something else altogether? What lesson might children learn when they are spanked for hitting, for example? Perhaps they learn that physical violence is okay if you are big or in charge; or that it's okay to hit boys, but not girls; or, perhaps, that it's okay for someone to hit them, but not okay for them to hit other people. Kids search out a way to make their own sense of the reality of the situation, regardless of what we wish to teach or what we say we are trying to impart.

Discipline will get the desired message across when parents are emotionally regulated and when the messages are unambiguous, in terms of both language and parental behavior. To this end, an essential aspect of good discipline is the development of clear family rules, warm responsiveness when children follow the rules, and consistent, calmly applied limit setting when rules are broken. This process allows room for trial-and-error learning and permits children to experiment safely. When this stance toward teaching is practiced, children discover that behavior problems do not mean that they are bad children but rather that they need to get back on track.

Research indicates that the best learning occurs within safe and trusting attachments (Brazelton & Greenspan, 2001; Langer, 2016; Schore, 2012; Shonkoff et al., 2012). When the heart of parenting has been honored, the work of parenting is easier. Children who feel secure in their relationship with their parents are confident that even if they break the rules and there are consequences, the attachment with their parents remains solid and secure (Siegel, 2020; Siegel & Hartzell, 2013). Like all of us, they will win some and lose some, and they will learn from mistakes. Within trusting attachments, children feel loved throughout the learning process.

Children can gain a sense of security and pride from learning and respecting family rules and boundaries. They like to know that their adults are paying attention and keeping the family on track. On the other hand, when behavior problems go unchecked, children can feel anxious or out of control. Children who don't learn to manage their behavior are likely to have issues in other relationships with teachers and peers, which can raise feelings of insecurity and self-doubt (Brazelton & Greenspan, 2001; Schore, 2015; Middlebrooks & Audage, 2008).

Learning and discipline directly address the last of children's 7 essential attachment needs: boundaries and structure. Healthy boundaries and structure are integral to the other six essential needs: safety and security, soothing, attunement, reliability, encouragement, and stimulation. Secure family relationships allow for optimal communication, learning, and the development of self-discipline. The approach that parents take to teaching and discipline will influence their children throughout their lives (Brazelton & Sparrow, 2006; Medina, 2014; Nakazawa, 2015; Middlebrooks & Audage, 2008; Schore, 2017; Shonkoff et al., 2012; van der Kolk, 2015).

SETTING LIMITS: HOW MUCH FREEDOM?

Adults continually make decisions about whether or not to restrict children's freedom. Children must learn restraint and to sacrifice some freedoms if the goal is for them to be functional, independent, contributing members of society who can enjoy their relational lives and raise the next generation of healthy humans. Limit setting is the action step for building this skill.

Parents make their own decisions about when and where to set boundaries. Therapists need a light touch in intervening, as there are numerous healthy ways to structure children's lives. Teachers and other caregivers also decide what boundaries they will set. So how do adults determine which limits to set—what freedoms the child should sacrifice? For parents, the decision is usually based on a mix of factors, including their histories, personal values, societal expectations, parent needs, and children's temperaments. Children also have opinions on the limits they will accept on their freedom. This is a two-way process, even though power is not equal between parents and children.

The 1960s Marshmallow Experiment illustrates the importance of developing personal restraint. Stanford University's Walter Mischel looked specifically at whether children's ability to delay gratification predicts future behavior or success (Mischel, 1958, 2014; Mischel & Shoda, 1988; Shoda et al., 1990). In this study, children between the ages of 4 and 6 years were given one marshmallow and told that the researcher was going to leave the room for 15 minutes. The children could choose whether to eat the marshmallow now and only get the one, or wait until the researcher returned and get a second marshmallow to eat. This study found that children who were able to delay gratification had better life outcomes across multiple areas, including success in social and academic settings. Although there is some debate on the interpretations of this study, the benefits of self-restraint are evident across similar findings.

ROLE MODELS: ACTIONS SPEAK LOUDER THAN WORDS

Parents also sacrifice some personal freedom in order to secure a place in their social groups, work lives, and larger society. Parents offer role modeling in the area of self-discipline by balancing autonomy and freedom while relinquishing some freedoms for a longer-term goal or the larger social good. Parents also sacrifice and exercise restraint when they prioritize caring for family members, nurturing friendships, maintaining healthy lifestyle habits, and balancing work and fun.

These are all examples for children. As role models, parents teach children how to behave in relationships, how to manage feelings, and how to cope with stress. It is what they do, rather than what they say, that provides information for their children.

ROLE MODELING "TOO BUSY"

Years ago, I was preparing my family to leave for a vacation. It was lunchtime, and I was busy packing, too busy to sit down and eat. I had on my mental checklist that the family should eat lunch before we left. My husband and son were eating, but my 7-year-old daughter was playing in her room. We called her repeatedly; no response.

Finally, I stopped what I was doing and went to talk with her. "I want you to eat now, so that we can leave soon," I said.

"Mom, I'm *too busy* to sit down and eat lunch," she answered.

Oh, my mirror. I was modeling *too busy*—no wonder she was ignoring our invitations to eat. I changed my stance and told her, "We are active women! I think we should take a break and go eat lunch before we leave for our trip." She immediately stopped what she was doing and we sat down for lunch.

K. S.

Children learn automatically through observation and experience, without having to think about it (Brazelton & Greenspan, 2001; Cozolino, 2014; Lester & Sparrow, 2010; Schore, 2015; Siegel, 2020). Verbal lessons require more mental work to process—especially if the lessons are contradictory to what the child is observing and experiencing.

ATTACHMENT, LEARNING, AND DISCIPLINE

In learning and discipline, attachment matters. Effectiveness at teaching and disciplining depends upon the extent to which parents have a sound, positively bonded relationship with their children (Langer, 2016; Taffel & Blau, 2002). Kids need to feel safely attached to adults to learn from them. As providers help parents explore ways to strengthen the home environment to create security, they facilitate those parents' ability to discipline and teach their children.

In session, therapists provide role modeling to contribute to the creation of a safe base for families. Therapists' attitudes and moods shape the feelings of security in the sessions, build the therapeutic relationship, and influence clients' learning. Does the provider feel emotionally robust or overly anxious? Is the therapist optimistic or discouraged? Families in crisis need a hopeful and secure base to help them stabilize.

Providers help parents create security as they foster it in the therapeutic relationship. Remember that treatment energy and resources flow downstream: to be stable and present, therapists must meet their own needs and prepare for their work mindfully. Even when this preparation is unseen by clients, it serves to model the stability and reliability we hope to instill in parents and children.

12

Ideal Scenarios: Optimal Teaching and Discipline

Good discipline is a mix of thoughtful preparation and creative flexibility, and it occurs in the context of a secure connection. Parents cannot anticipate when discipline will be required or what issues will arise. It is more of a messy art than a science, often practiced on the move. As a result, regardless of good intentions, efforts at discipline are often the product of impulses in the moment.

Children's need for discipline is not always conveniently timed. Whether it is in a grocery line, at a party, in a car, or at the end of a tiring day, discipline is often exercised when parents are not their best selves. Especially challenging times for discipline are bedtime, when parents and children are tired; transitional times, such as afterschool hours when the family is coming together and not yet settled; or times when family members are sick, stressed, hungry, busy, and not emotionally regulated.

Family therapists can help parents prepare ahead of time for the inevitably stressful times when it is so easy for them to be inconsistent or impulsive. That is why it is crucial for parents to work in advance to clarify their priorities and expectations, and to prepare to be mindful of their feelings when practicing discipline. A primary aspect of thoughtful parenting is finding a way to adhere to the game plan: to remain aligned with their parenting intentions. Even in the heat of the moment, parents are capable of deciding what to focus on, and of choosing their attitude and their responses. It is the job of the family therapist to facilitate this process.

ELEMENTS OF GOOD DISCIPLINE

Some parents resist the idea of firm discipline, thinking they don't want their children to be obedient little soldiers. These parents do have a point; many children who are well behaved are not regulated—they are afraid. Therapists can explore this anxiety and clarify with parents that the mindless or anxious compliance they fear is not the result of healthy discipline, but rather the result of parenting gone awry. Parental rigidity and intolerance lead to child fear and loss of spontaneity. On the contrary, healthy discipline fosters trust, good judgment, self-efficacy, and self-control. Some critical life skills develop through childhood experiences of clear boundaries and expectations; among them are behavioral self-control, social skills, self-confidence, the ability to apply effort toward goals, and frustration tolerance.

What is healthy discipline? It is clear, consistent, not harsh or shaming, and applied by thoughtful parents with empathy for their children's vulnerabilities and immature emotional systems. Children, and even teens, have immature neurological systems that are not ready to regulate through the situations and feelings they face (Porges, 2011; Schore, 2017; Siegel, 2015, 2020). Throughout childhood and adolescence, they need the parental container (with clear limits and boundaries) to help them make safe choices. Children need to learn when to slow down, when to stop, and when it is time to get moving again. Semimature adolescents especially need mature guidance as they move through new levels of autonomy in decision making.

To create a culture of healthy discipline, we recommend therapists focus on fostering the following requirements for a *healthy learning environment* (which are compatible with the 7 essential attachment needs):

- Security and truthworthiness
- Reliably positive responses to children's successes

- Clear and consistent expectations (structure)
- Emotionally regulated adults
- Adults who do not overreact to problems
- Consequences are low in intensity and lack any inadvertent relational reward

Secure, Trustworthy, and Positive Environments

Security is an essential part of good discipline and a prerequisite for learning. Adults can best influence and teach children in the context of a positive and trusting relationship. The more attuned parents are to their children, the more the children's brains light up with activity and readiness for learning. To effectively teach, parents must connect before they correct.

Remember that discipline is not punishment, but teaching. A child cannot be taught when they are not open to learning: when they are not calm and receptive, and when they do not have a sense of safety, trust, and attunement with their caregivers. When discipline does not serve to shift behaviors, it is usually because this foundation has not been set or has been disrupted.

When a person feels safe and secure, their brain is in a peaceful and integrated state. In this state, receptivity is higher, and children are better able to explore. They are more flexible, open, and curious. Not only does the trusting relationship with children light up their brains, it also motivates them to maintain a positive connection with their parents.

When a person is threatened or feels unsafe, they are in a limbic or sympathetic state where they are more defensive and concerned with survival. This state is not a learning state; it is an anxious or angry state. In a stressful parent–child relationship, children are not ready for learning. At a biological level, conflict causes the release of stress hormones like cortisol and adrenaline, which interfere with learning and social connection. Over time, these stress hormones can interfere with brain development (Carrion & Wong, 2012; Kiecolt-Glaser et al., 2010; Langer, 2016; Middlebrooks & Audage, 2008; Shonkoff et al., 2012; Snyder et al., 2011; Teicher et al., 2003; Todeschin et al., 2009).

An essential feature of creating safety is a steady state of awareness and appreciation of children's successes. When people feel seen and appreciated, they feel more confident and redouble their efforts to repeat successes. Helping parents focus on noticing and articulating what their children are already doing well is an impactful way to increase trust in the relationship and encourage positive behavior.

Creating a trustworthy environment does not mean the atmosphere is always harmonious, but rather that there is safety and understanding even when conflict emerges. Adults are bigger, stronger, and kind. They can be counted on to weather conflict with steadiness. A productive stance for a parent is to acknowledge their inherent power and manifest it firmly but gently.

Clear and Consistent Expectations

Another component of healthy discipline is the creation of an environment that is clear and predictable. Predictable routines and structure are often overlooked as beneficial elements of child behavior management. When these concepts are applied, the home is similar day to day; for example, meals are at the same time, bedtime routines are unvarying, and children know when to do homework. Letting the routine slip for special occasions or holidays is okay for normally developing children, but for highly anxious kids, or any children struggling to cope, it should be avoided whenever possible. Such stability reduces demands on the child and helps them remain calm and make sense of their world.

Of course, many sturdy children can tolerate schedule variation, and some even crave change. Thus, consistency should be dependent on the child's personal need for stability. Wherever children are struggling emotionally or behaviorally, increasing structure and reducing demands is the first path of intervention, with the end goal of supporting them in reestablishing equilibrium.

One way children learn lessons is by identifying and repeating patterns; the more consistent the pattern, the easier this is to do. A familiar structure reduces stress and helps children organize and control their behavior because they do not need to try to figure out what comes next. It is easier to decode expectations when the environment is structured and clear.

Changes in structure are sometimes unavoidable; for more fragile children, give advance notice of changes in routine whenever possible. If children rely heavily on routines to maintain their stability, try helping parents create a daily schedule that children can see. Break the day into blocks that are marked with activities and responsibilities; even label free time. When an unexpected change occurs, parents can write "oops" on a sticky note along with the new activity for that time and stick it on the schedule. This often helps highly sensitive children adjust to inconsistency. It is a step toward the goal of increasing comfort with change—building flexibility and acceptance of life's inevitable variations.

Adult Emotional Regulation: Eliminating Overreactions

When adults are emotionally regulated, they are more able to respond with consistency. If parents' reactions are the same each time, children do not have to wonder what they might do. When children try out a new behavior, the more consistent parents' responses are to that behavior, the more quickly children will learn. With consistency in adult response, positive behavior takes root more quickly and misbehavior is more quickly abandoned. However, if parents respond to the behavior in a variety of ways, they actually extend the life of any misbehavior as children work to figure out which response it will bring. The children of predictable parents know what to expect.

This is why adult regulation matters with discipline. Without it, a parent can respond impulsively or emotionally to misbehavior, which inadvertently undercuts their attempts to stop that behavior. Erratic discipline—giving a time-out at home, scolding when out in public, sending the child to his room when friends visit, and ignoring the problem altogether when the father is tired—creates confusion. This inconsistent pattern is called *intermittent reinforcement*: the behavior is sometimes discouraged and other times is allowed or reinforced.

Intermittent reinforcement is the most robust reinforcement schedule. It increases the likelihood of the child repeating the unwanted behavior because the child never knows if the behavior will be met with a reward, or not. This inadvertently encourages continued testing. Intermittently reinforced behavior is tough to change.

Another ill effect of adult dysregulation is a tendency to overreact, which can lead to parental harshness and explosiveness. Overreaction can also occur if a parent believes the best way to halt a behavior is a very large response. In either case, the overreaction overwhelms their child's nervous system. Harsh punishments or an out-of-control adult damage the trust and safety required for a secure relationship and optimal learning. When adult regulation is adequate, discipline is more successful and less traumatic. Adult regulation is a requisite element of good discipline. Learning to do this is difficult and some of the hardest work of parenting.

Winning the Long Game

Punitive responses to children's behavioral missteps are part of many parenting approaches, and parents often incorrectly believe that the more substantial and aversive the consequence, the more effective it will be. The problem with this strategy is that excessive focus on consequences can overtake parenting, placing undue attention and passion on punishment. This negativity can ultimately damage the parent–child relationship and alienate children.

In working with parents, therapists can suggest the approach of prioritizing the *long game* over the *short game* in child-rearing. The short game is dealing with behavior at that moment, influencing the child to stop hitting or to do her homework. The long game is the maintenance of a healthy, positive parent–child relationship, gradually building self-control and positive behavior. We emphasize winning the long game at all costs, even if it means temporarily losing the short game.

This plays out via parents setting a limit every single time a rule is broken, but never doing so in a damaging way: no yelling, no insulting, no spanking, no adult dysregulation. While this sounds permissive to some, the key to its success is that limit setting is never skipped over. It is consistent and reliably applied, with no drama. No rule breaking is ever overlooked. In this model the limit setting is matter-of-fact and not harsh—not driven by parents' intense emotions. And limits are not set with the toxin of adult negativity. To win the long game we must be able to be patient in the midst of misbehavior and to sometimes sacrifice immediate satisfaction.

BUSINESS AND PERSONAL SIDES OF PARENTING

Another way to think about the consistency and positivity that create the most effective parenting style is to draw from Jaime Raser's (2003) description of parenting as having a *business side* and a *personal side*.

The business side can be described as highly structured, consisting of limits, rules, education, schedule, and discipline. These are the building blocks of clarity, consistency, and stability, which are required for children to understand expectations and be tutored in the practical ways of the world.

The personal side can be described as nurturing and includes play, fun, cuddling, love, respect, caring, socializing, friendship, and empathic connection. It is the touchy-feely side of parenting and provides critical elements for building self-awareness, emotional well-being, and social competence.

Ideal parenting balances and separates the business and personal sides of the relationship. When these aspects of parenting are in balance, children are raised with structure and discipline, but also warmth and compassion. When these sides are out of balance, parenting can be overly strict and restrictive or overly permissive and lax.

Children who are challenging can often trigger overcompensation in one direction or another. Parents may err on the side of "all he needs is a lot of love" and overfocus on the personal, or they may strongly react to misbehavior and overfocus on the business side. Friends and family members may see children's misbehavior and comment about lack of discipline, pressing the parents to become more rigid and authoritarian.

In actuality, all children benefit from a balance of the business and personal sides of parenting; challenging children require high levels of both. They need both high structure and high nurturance to thrive. The business side provides structure in the form of a solid routine, clear rules, and predictable limit setting. The personal side provides high nurturance in the form of frequent, accurate, sincere recognitions, and takes judicious care to avoid energizing negative behaviors.

The business and personal sides of parenting should be crisply distinguished from one another. Setting a limit is not a personal comment about the child; it is just a behavioral limit. Similarly, business side structure does not need to take over moments of fun and affection. Spontaneity can coexist with firmly held limits.

When the business and personal sides of parenting are blurred, problems often occur. Interpreting children's failure to follow the rules as a lack of respect or taking children's misbehavior personally is blurring the boundaries. At these times, parents may allow their feelings to drive their parenting decisions. Where they feel disrespected or attacked by their children, they might respond with an intense emotional outburst or withdraw from the interaction altogether. In either case, the parents' emotional reaction can lead to an inability to deal effectively with misbehavior. In these circumstances, limit setting will be much less effective due to either overemphasizing children's errors with a passionate, emotion-laden response or by disempowering parents who are no longer holding limits. This blurring results in less clear, concise, matter-of-fact limit setting.

Another type of blurring occurs when parents allow the business side to intrude on the personal side. For example, parents might be overly rigid and insist children play a game a certain way or might enforce arbitrary rules without taking children's feelings into account. Where parents let the business side of parenting intrude into personal time with their children, they may overstructure and overcontrol what could be a spontaneous, creative, mutually satisfying time together, robbing themselves and their children of attuned connection. Having time for business and pleasure is as important for adults as it is for children.

EFFECTIVE DISCIPLINE BEGINS WITH RESPONSIVE PARENTING

Responsive parenting means parents consciously choosing their behaviors in relationship with their children rather than impulsively acting out—choosing to respond from the prefrontal cortex rather than reacting from the limbic system (Badenoch, 2008; Siegel, 2020). When parents are mindful, they can choose.

Responsive parenting requires a mindful stance. It requires being present in the moment, thoughtful, and accepting, holding an awareness of one's own emotions, thoughts, and intentions in addition to children's feelings, perspectives, and developmental stages. Responsive parents accept the whole child, the good and the bad. This does not mean glossing over conflict or ignoring problems, but facing both with an open heart and mind—a sensitive awareness that includes acceptance of every moment, including the moments that parents like and those that they do not. Such parents accept life's constellation of ever-shifting feelings and behaviors with equanimity. Mindfulness is a state of mind, an approach to life. This being said, adults go in and out of this state, and it is a learned skill to return to it when they default to nonmindful patterns—which everyone does when life is out of balance.

As therapists, you may observe parents who are already competent at maintaining moment-to-moment mindfulness and choicefulness within themselves. Rather than dwelling on how to stop a behavior they don't like, they take a more reflective stance: "Hmmm . . . something is going on here. How do I want to respond?" This involves parents entertaining more curiosity about the situation, prioritizing self-regulation before responding, and maintaining awareness of the child's developmental stage as they choose their response.

This process is another example of focusing on the long game of parenting rather than on immediate resolution of problematic behaviors. In the long game, parents focus intently on fostering the relationship with their children and on maintaining trust and connection, while the short game focuses on controlling behavior in the moment. From a stance of sensitivity and respect, parents are able to see past the behavior at hand.

Some parents are instinctively aware that winning the short game often comes at the cost of the long game, and that focusing on the short game is best attempted only after the long game is being won. A focus on the long game inspires parents to look past their children's moment-to-moment behaviors to see their true nature. Grounded in the long game, parents can hold a relational focus that makes it easier to honor children's points of view and to respect their inherent goodness and value. Even telling children "no" can be done in ways that foster, rather than damage, the relationship.

Mindful Responsivity

Responsive parents practice mindfully observing children's expressions, tone of voice, and body language to gather information about their experiences. Children may share their thoughts, feelings, and associations. To the degree that parents can recognize and honor these things, they build toward winning the long game—that is, a secure long-term relationship that is a solid foundation for effective discipline.

Mindful parenting does not mean that everything the child does is acceptable; instead, it means disciplining with love and respect and without judgment or criticism of who the child is as a person. Awareness of children's problems and weaknesses is also a part of mindful parenting: incorporating awareness of where the child needs to grow and change, honoring their pace, and trusting their natural drive for growth.

Acceptance of self is also a skill of the responsive parent. Parents are sometimes hardest on themselves and are often driven by internal and external messages extolling self-sacrifice and self-criticism transmitted from family, friends, and society. Where parents make an effort to practice self-acceptance and patience with themselves, they are more able to embody these qualities with their children. This stance is calming to the nervous systems of both parents and their children. It communicates security and patience and is an attachment-sound approach to parenting.

CHILDREN'S LEARNING: EMOTIONAL REGULATION MATTERS

Remember, discipline means teaching, and children learn best when the PNS (ventral vagal) is dominant—when they are in the rest-and-digest mode. The social engagement system, which is required for learning, is not functional when the body is in the SNS fight-or-flight mode (Levine, 2015; Porges, 2011, 2017; Siegel, 2020). Effective discipline requires facilitation of a sense of security and stability by calm, caring adults. When children feel safe and socially attached, their nervous systems can relax and regulate into the PNS-dominant state that facilitates learning.

Of course, well-functioning parents still have to manage dysregulated children. This is just a part of family life. But these parents are adept at realizing that children's dysregulation is not a prime moment for teaching (a topic we address further in Chapter 13). Dysregulated children are not making logical and purposeful choices or exhibiting intentionally or morally wrong behavior. They are operating out of an unintegrated, unstable state analogous to the behavior of a lizard running from a loud, threatening sound. When parents are effective and responsive, they respond to the dysregulated child in ways that stabilize that child's nervous system. They teach by setting limits on behavior firmly but calmly, and then quickly return to normal family life.

Learning and the Brain

Children are always learning. At a neurobiological level, learning occurs naturally as children's brains mature. As neurons myelinate, interconnect, and integrate, developing brains become more accurate, efficient, smart, and fast.

Remember that neurons that fire together wire together (Hebb's rule). This associative learning is enhanced when information is presented repeatedly. The more children repeat behaviors or thoughts, the more likely they are to become automatic. This is how consistent and predictable routines, responses, and limit setting foster learning: by creating repeated experiences that are easily encoded in the brain. Both bad habits and good habits are ingrained through practice. Habits can be altered in only one way: by repeating new behavior patterns.

Children learn at various levels. Sometimes those levels are explicit (processed with the hippocampus), higher brain, cortical learning; sometimes they are implicit (not involving such processing), primarily with the limbic system. Implicit learning occurs through the nervous system taking notice without integration into explicit factual or autobiographical memories. It can be associative (for example, when Dad has that look on his face, bad things happen) or skills-based (for example, adding "Please" increases chances of success). Ideally, children learn meaningful information on both explicit and implicit levels, so that the messages are more consolidated and deeply integrated into the brain.

When they think of teaching and discipline, adults usually think about explicit learning. Parents work to explicitly teach manners, self-control, and neatness. But explicit knowledge is the tip of the iceberg of what kids learn from adults; implicit learning is where a lot of the essential education occurs.

Implicit learning is often imparted unintentionally, and it is powerful. Implicit messages are their own form of learning, which can be either reinforced or sabotaged by explicit learning. When parents consciously try to teach self-control and also practice self-control at home, the implicit message is consistent with the expressed message. This alignment lends power and credence to the lesson. Implicit learning also stands alone, however. Adults' behaviors around children are potent forms of teaching that are often not intended to be lessons, but are taken in by children as learning. When things are going well, children learn many skills and interaction patterns implicitly. This implicit learning path is where children learn they are valuable and can trust others. They also learn that they are due respect, that their feelings matter, and that restraint is important.

13

Problem Scenarios: Dysfunction in Discipline

Discipline can go downhill for a thousand reasons. Every parent who comes into our offices has a unique struggle around teaching and discipline. Their struggles tend to result from patterns of thinking and reaction that are below their awareness. Parenting choices may not feel like choices, but rather unexamined responses that feel like the only way. Due to a fast-paced life, elevated stress, or personal history, parents can find themselves parenting on autopilot. External pressures to form the child in a certain way, or be a certain type of parent only further fuel frustration and rigidity. This can lead to a lack of perspective.

Once perspective is lost parents can slip into negative patterns that cause them to lose at the long game of maintaining relationship. A cycle of child struggles and ineffective parenting often emerges. This only increases stress in the family system. Highly stressed parents may overfocus on the business or the personal side of parenting, interacting in ways that are overly rigid and controlling or excessively permissive and laid back. Either inclination can contribute to a weakness in the secure parent–child relationship and undermine consistency. This tension sets families up to lose at both the short and the long game.

Rather than making a laundry list of potential discipline problems and strategies for addressing them, we describe categories of parenting problems in broad strokes to help you as a therapist focus your attention and crack the code on where to target parenting interventions.

IDENTIFYING DISCIPLINE PROBLEMS

Discipline problems are likely to occur when parents are inconsistent, emotionally unstable, or disconnected. Recall the *elements of a healthy learning environment* (Chapter 12): (1) security and trust; (2) reliably positive responses to children's successes; (3) clear and consistent expectations (structure); (4) emotionally regulated adults; (5) adults who do not overreact to problems; and (6) consequences are low in intensity and lack any inadvertent relational reward. Inconsistency, emotional instability, or disconnection all impact parents' ability to build the kind of learning environment that is conducive to effective discipline.

These are not discrete categories. Positive patterns in one often overlap or fuel success in another. Similarly, in more troublesome circumstances, problems in one area often contribute to difficulties in another. For efficiency's sake, we discuss potential discipline problems involving each of these elements as separate dynamics, categorizing them as issues of parental inconsistency, emotional instability, and disconnection.

Inconsistency

Inconsistency in parenting arises when parents lack the ability or will to clarify their intentions and structure their family environment. Unclear expectations for the parents and children mean that structure is absent and parental guidance erratic. Children don't know what to expect and, in the absence of predictable patterns and rhythms, have more trouble regulating and organizing themselves.

Inconsistent parenting can be identified by:

- Chaotic schedules, poor organization
- Absence of rules
- Ever-shifting rules based on parental mood, whims, or energy level
- Erratic rule enforcement
- Consequences and rewards applied some times, not others
- Excessive freedom for children

Parents with inconsistent patterns are likely to be disorganized in sessions. They tend to struggle to follow through on plans or to stick with topics to their conclusion. Their attendance at appointments may be erratic. They may disregard the need for structure, stating that they don't see the point, and may speak of the fear of oppressing or overpowering their children if they were to enact stronger structure. Their children may seem not to know what's going on and may run wild or test limits often, with parents responding with inconsistent or absent holding of limits in the waiting room or therapy office.

Emotional Instability

In families with emotionally unstable parents, adults fail to regulate their own emotional states. Parents are more likely to be easily dysregulated when they have had difficult childhoods, suffer from mental health disorders, are involved in substance abuse, or are under high stress; some may simply not have learned the importance of emotional steadiness when raising children.

A particularly destructive result of lack of parental regulation is highly dramatic responses to negativity and problem behaviors. Intense adverse reactions to children's errors or misbehaviors cause undue stress in the short term and can inadvertently create a negative identity for children in the long term.

Emotionally unstable parents can be identified by:

- Focus on their own emotional state over that of their children
- Tendency to take children's behavior personally
- Attempts to control situations and their children through domination, threats, or outbursts
- Misconception that bigger consequences produce bigger changes
- Chaotic home environment (common in cases with substance abuse or family violence)
- Lack of awareness when their behavior is inappropriate or hurtful
- Presence of abusive behavior

Parenting behaviors or interactions to watch for with emotional instability include strong focus on punishments, which can be harsh, or a focus of therapy on parental frustration, fear, or anger. Emotionally unstable parents are easily overwhelmed and are intense and passionate in their interactions with the therapist. They may name-call or label their children as bad. Children from these environments may discuss or play out fear of their parents' reactions.

Disconnection

Unfortunately, parent–child disconnection is prevalent in our rushed and pressured society. Families can overlook a critical component of family life, parent–child connection, merely due to rushing and busyness. They may prioritize lessons and responsibilities to such a degree that they impinge on their relationships, or drift away from connection without awareness of what they are giving up. Other families are at heightened risk for shallow relationships due to the parents' histories and patterns. When disconnection is an issue in a family, there is often an absence of security and trustworthiness at home and a lack of authentic positivity toward children.

Disconnection can be identified by:

- Lack of parental emotional awareness or sensitivity
- Lack of attunement to children
- Disinterest or lack of focus on children's experiences and internal life
- Inability to see what is beautiful and valuable in children (sometimes presents as indictment of children)
- Unrealistic expectations
- Lack of compassion and attunement

Parenting behaviors or interactions to watch for as clues to disconnection include parents often talking over or failing to listen to children. They may override children's perceptions and opinions. There may be physical distance, diminished eye contact, and an absence of comfortable touch; excessive complaining about children, possibly in front of them; and a general insensitivity to children in sessions. Parents may fail to play with their children, instead showing up as overly logical, judgmental, and task focused. A domineering, disconnected parent will display low listening and high direction, while a disinterested disconnected parent will display both low listening and low direction.

As the therapist recognizes parenting patterns that disrupt effective discipline for individual families, the best plan for helping becomes more clear. Parents who are more inconsistent may benefit from an emphasis on interventions that help them more sturdily enact the business side of parenting and separate it from the personal side. Emotionally unstable parents may need a stronger lean into emotion management, and disconnected parents will need to be grounded in the importance of connected, attuned, and mindful parenting.

HIGH ROAD/LOW ROAD: THE IMPORTANCE OF PARENT EMOTIONAL REGULATION

When adults are emotionally calm, centered, and alert, they are better at everything, including parenting. It is when they are stressed, tired, or otherwise disoriented that parents are more likely to regret what they say or do. They are vulnerable to the same disconnection from their prefrontal cortices as children—a disconnection from Dan Siegel's Nine Control Functions (attention, empathy, intuition, morality, flexibility, reduced fear, attunement, and physical and emotional regulation)—in response to adrenaline and cortisol overload (Siegel, 2020, 2017).

Attributes held by the prefrontal cortex—including highest-order thinking, self-soothing, ethical decision making, generosity, and putting things in perspective—are necessary for making good parenting decisions in tough situations. Adults need to engage this part of their brain to make wise decisions and be compassionate with others. It might not be surprising to learn that drinking alcohol or using other drugs can impair prefrontal cortex function.

One useful framework for describing parents' state of regulation is Siegel's *high road/low road* metaphor (Siegel, 2015; Figure 13.1). When parents are

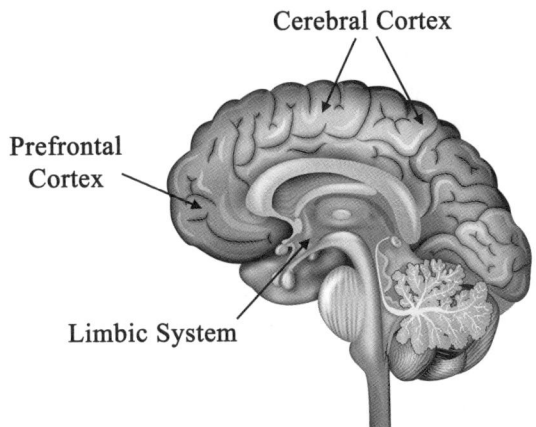

Figure 13.1   The Vertical Brain: High and Low Road in the Brain
SOURCE: © Gunita Reine/Depositphotos.com

using their higher-order thinking, they are on the high road. On the high road, parents are emotionally balanced and aware, in a state of mental integration, and able to use their nine control functions. When parents are under the influence of negative forces such as fatigue, anger, fear, or shame, they are more vulnerable to sliding down to the low road, where they are more reactive and emotionally driven (Byrne, 2019; Davidson & McEwen, 2012; McGreevy, 2011; Siegel, 2020; Wilson, 2013). They are no longer putting things in perspective, being aware, or being compassionate.

Parents are not perfect; they alternate between the high and low roads. When they inevitably veer toward the low road, they may not be conscious of the shift in mindset, as being emotionally activated reduces self-awareness. A parent who is traveling the low road is likely to make the error of yelling, threatening, overindulging, or giving up. They may even shut down and feel unable to take any action. Mindfulness, patience, and humility are not accessible to parents on the low road. This path often leads to mistakes and regret.

During heightened conflict, communication between parent and child can become intensely charged. It is the adult's responsibility to remain on the high road in those moments. If adults lose control or fly off the handle when they are upset with children, a teachable moment is lost, and the adult's dysregulation can quickly catapult children into a similarly dysregulated state. When children are flooded with emotional distress, it is easy but ineffective to join their turmoil. What children need in those moments is a regulated parent. Adults are bigger and stronger, and it is their responsibility to be wiser and calmer than children (Baylin & Hughes, 2016; Schore, 2015; Siegel & Bryson, 2012).

To model is to teach. Role modeling is a significant factor in discipline and helping children learn to manage tough emotions. How parents manage their intense emotions serves as examples to their children. How do parents manage their anger, frustration, and weariness? Whatever parents do is an implicit endorsement of their children doing the same. When adults can understand and manage their feelings and behavior, they set a standard for children to do the same. A parent who is telling children to manage their anger must also model anger control to be effective. When parents take care of their own business, emotionally and socially, everyone in the family benefits, not just the parents.

NOT A TEACHABLE MOMENT

Parents spend a lot of time trying to teach their children. They work to teach them to say "please," to put their dirty clothes in the hamper, not to hit, and so much more. And most parents have found this teaching more difficult than expected. "It's simple! Just put your clothes in the hamper, not on the floor! Why is it so hard?" There are loads of reasons why this can be so tough; the reason we want to emphasize here is timing.

Parents—and most others—tend to try to teach lessons when things are going wrong. When do they give their child a talk about saying "please"? Right after the child skips saying it. When do parents remind children to put clothes in the hamper? When they see children throwing their clothes, infuriatingly, on the floor . . . again. And naturally, they want to teach their children not to hit when the child just walloped his brother.

This pattern of teaching what to do instead is natural for humans. The human eye sees keenly what is not right; adults are acculturated to notice what is wrong and take steps to correct it. While this is natural, it doesn't work very well for teaching. At the moment when parents are most motivated to teach, children are the least able or motivated to learn. As discussed in detail in previous chapters, the reasons for this are biological: When a child is "in trouble," this reads as a danger signal to the child's nervous system. Adrenaline and cortisol production are triggered, and the SNS overtakes the PNS. The sense of calmness and security necessary for social engagement, good judgment, perspective taking, and learning is replaced by a defensive state of fight, flight, or faint. The immature brain of a child, with its underdeveloped prefrontal cortex, is less able to remain attentive, logical, and cooperative in the best of times; when in a defensive SNS state, this ability is further weakened.

In behavioral terms, a child who is in an SNS-predominant state may respond to parental correction with arguing, screaming, avoiding, withdrawing, defying, or lying. They do so because in that moment, they are emotional and reactive and not in a responsive learning state.

So, when we sweetly tell children they are making mistakes, doing it wrong, and need to stop, they may take this as helpful guidance, or they may take it as being picked on. We all know from experience which interpretation is most likely. If they feel nagged, criticized, or challenged, they experience emotional stress, a form of threat, and become defensive—perhaps in a minor way (irritated and uncomfortable), or perhaps in a major way (defensive, enraged, feeling attacked).

It doesn't matter that these corrections come from loving parents who are reminding them for their own good. All parents have experienced the fruitless struggle of trying to correct children who are upset and not the least bit interested in being told they are wrong. Not only are these efforts to teach experienced as harsh and critical—even when we do our best to come across gently—but they tend to occur in moments when children are not receptive at all.

Parents in this situation know they are no real threat to their children, so they can be stunned by the intensity of the resistance to even kind corrections. But the children's base brain and vagal system respond instinctively, triggered by the sense of being opposed. They feel provoked. Once parents understand this context, it is clear that the best learning does not occur through nagging or correction. The most relaxed and most natural learning occurs when children are in an integrated brain state, calm and secure. Parents can learn to create and sustain this state of mind, and that it's not complicated to do so.

Teach parents that they can and should correct misbehavior—but to do so mildly, without investing energy in that moment, which is unlikely to be a learning moment. When parents see misbehavior, have them offer a succinct correction in as low-key a manner as possible. For example: if their child hits, they should state, "No hitting," in an unruffled way. When adults are calm and not lecturing, raising their voices, or threatening, they avoid activating children's defensive brains and so are less likely to trigger defiance, tears, or tantrums. Keep in mind, however, that even this style of gentle and mild correction, while necessary, is not the moment of most powerful learning; it is not a teachable moment.

To create teachable moments, we take steps to keep children feeling safe and their brains in an integrated state so that learning can occur. We recommend using NHA to accomplish this, resolutely not giving excessive attention or reaction to missteps, and commending children for all accomplishments, even tiny ones. This style may feel silly at first, but it promotes a sense of safety and is nourishing. Finding and celebrating children's successes throughout the day creates feelings of pride, achievement, and joy in children—the stuff from which teachable moments are made. Parental emotional regulation is a prerequisite for successfully implementing this approach.

DEGREES OF DISCONNECTION: HEALTHY AND NOT

Parents typically experience varying levels of connection and disconnection with their children as they shift between closeness, distance, and back again. These shifts are natural in the relationship and are usually not harmful.

Rifts are inevitable in all connections. Even the most mindful and regulated parents will create ruptures in the parent–child relationship. A certain amount of disconnection can occur when limits are set with children, since limits go against their immediate drive or desire. Saying "no" to someone can create distance, though it is essential for setting boundaries. It should not communicate a rejection of the child or the relationship; it is a rejection of the behavior only.

Parent–child disconnection can play out in three different ways that are relevant to our discussion. In the best circumstances, the parents accept and understand the ebb and flow of closeness, allow discord to occur, and reconnect with children as soon as possible. This scenario is ideal and wise. However, when things go awry in families, parents tend to react in less productive ways.

Some parents react negatively to feelings of disconnection, fearing they are rejecting or mistreating their children. They may feel shaken or hurt by the disruption, or take it personally, fearing loss of relationship with their children. These parents may then avoid setting limits. Permissive parenting is a common outcome of this avoidance of conflict.

In other families, when the discipline practiced is harsh or repair is absent, the disconnect can become chronic, even toxic. Children may end up feeling rejected or humiliated as parents remain distant over extended periods. This pattern can lead children to feel embarrassed, guilty, or ashamed. A lack of sensitivity to children's feelings of vulnerability or failure to repair can lead to self-criticism, feelings of worthlessness, and hopelessness in the child (Tronick, 2007).

It is important to note, and what often goes unacknowledged, is that the best discipline occurs in relationship—and the practice of discipline does not require a relational rupture. If limit setting is practiced thoughtfully and predictably, the parent–child relationship can be tolerant of limit setting. And, the benefits of clear boundaries can be reaped.

CHILDREN'S EMBARRASSMENT, GUILT, AND SHAME

In all the problematic parenting patterns described in this chapter—unstable, disconnected, and emotionally dysregulated—critical, judging, or demeaning language can make things worse. Therapists should guide parents in understanding that words are powerful, and that the language they use can instill deep feelings of embarrassment, guilt, or shame in children. These are distinct feelings with different psychological triggers and consequences:

- *Embarrassment* is a feeling of discomfort and self-consciousness in reaction to one's behavior due to imagined or real negative judgments by others. Children are very susceptible to embarrassment; corrections that must occur in public should be made with as little display as possible to avoid harm.
- *Guilt* is an emotional reaction to the belief that one has broken a personal moral code, and results in feelings of regret or in disappointment in the self. This feeling of guilt might be resolved by making amends, such as making an effort to fix the wrong done. The misery of guilt may drive a person to seek repair and help them learn to avoid such transgressions in the future. Where parents gently guide children through the repair process, they can recover from guilt.
- *Shame* is a deeper feeling of disgrace, dishonor, or humiliation, which can result in children hiding or withdrawing from others. Shame is an innate emotional response to violating a social expectation or norm. It can be triggered by one's social awareness or feedback from others. It is a socially based experience that can lead to fear of rejection or social isolation. Where guilt results in a bad feeling about the behavior, shame is more likely to create a bad feeling about the self. Shame is potentially more damaging to self-esteem over time. Children can recover from shame and feel connected and accepted through positive, supportive interactions with the primary people in their lives.

Toxic Shame

Toxic shame, as described by Allan Schore (2015), is children's experience of chronic rejection or constant criticism by adults. This pattern can be created in families where parents are always angry, severely neglectful, or hold children in disdain. When children feel a sense of rejection or absolute disconnection from parents, they can internalize it as loneliness and worthlessness.

Feelings of self-loathing and hopelessness can result if children are left without the experience of positive connection and repair. Shame and self-rejection can lead to chronic anxiety or depression, which can impair the healthy development of the brain, body, and emotional systems. Repair from toxic shame requires that children have a safe and responsive home where they can recover, learn, and grow.

Parents should never use shame on purpose, nor should they induce shame through harsh reactions or punishment—no matter what the child has done. Discipline should not involve humiliation, name-calling, sustained anger, or rejection of children. Instead, the focus should be on learning, boundaries, respect, and collaboration. This is best established by reconnecting with children after a dispute, allowing them to make amends for mistakes, and embracing them into the family after misbehavior.

Children can feel vulnerable during conflict or when parents set limits, so degrading language cuts deeply. While it is true that guilt, shame, and embarrassment may alter children's behavior, it is at a robust negative cost to their self-esteem, and also to the parent–child relationship (Schore, 2001, 2015; Siegel & Bryson, 2012; Tronick, 2007, 2017). Children need to trust that adults are there to boost them up, not tear them down—to encourage, not discourage, their growth.

When such ruptures have occurred in the parent–child relationship, it is the parent's job to sensitively seek reconnection and repair. Therapists can assist parents in practicing attuned reconnection and repair with their children. If parents have not experienced this type of repair in past relationships, they may welcome specific discussion on when and how to pursue reconnection and repair.

14

Treatment Interventions: Transforming Families by Transforming Discipline

Effective discipline is not just another item on a parent's daily checklist. It is a parental lifestyle—built into the moment-to-moment relationship between parents and children, not just turned on when problems occur. It is continually being established and acted on, even when there is no problem in sight. A transformational disciplinary approach is part of the fabric of daily relationships and grows out of a profound grasp and acceptance of children. It is a new way of life, and it can change everything.

In this chapter, we offer a comprehensive perspective that steers clear of seeing discipline as just a way to correct problem behaviors. It is easy for therapists to be drawn into focusing our work with children and families on managing problematic behaviors; indeed, problems are usually the reason parents seek our support in parenting their children. To be truly transformational, we need to have the vision and spine to resist buying into the paradigm that treatment is about children's problems and bad behavior. Instead, we hold that the endgame of effective discipline is raising children with the self-efficacy and self-regulation required to live out their highest capabilities. We maintain this stance firmly, even when discussing discipline.

At the root of effective discipline is the parent's responsibility to create an optimal environment for learning. We know that when children feel secure, loved, valued, and on-track in their relationship with their parents (rather than judged, criticized, or pressured), their brains are calm and integrated: open to change. They have access to higher-order functions such as logic, attention, and cooperation. This is when children are ready for learning and where dysfunctional patterns can be transformed.

Implied in this perspective is that therapists can also only effectively teach parents when parents feel safe and calm. Traditional psychotherapy practices of listening, reflecting, and witnessing are vital in creating this secure environment. Once parents are relaxed, psychoeducation can begin. So therapists can start all parenting work by engaging the parents in a way that produces a sense of safety and acceptance.

Here, we revisit the Nurtured Heart Approach, a set of strategies that supports parents in predictably creating a warm, positive, appreciative home environment. Therapists can use the same approach when working with young clients.

TAKE ADVANTAGE OF TEACHABLE MOMENTS: THE SECOND STAND OF NHA

Therapists working to transform families can begin by exploring with parents ways to interact with children that create a calm and open learning state. It is valuable for parents to understand that they are instrumental in creating this state of mind, and that doing so is feasible.

Recall the 3 Stands of the Nurtured Heart Approach:

Stand 1: Absolutely No—Adults do not respond to misbehavior with particular focus, passion, or attentiveness. They are careful to not reward problems with a big reaction or give the impression that problem behaviors lead to a greater relational connection.

Stand 2: Absolutely Yes—Adults recognize and appreciate anything positive in the child's behaviors, efforts, attitudes, character traits. They work to see the child principally in terms of the child's assets and virtues, and to articulate this to the child.

Stand 3: Absolutely Clear—Adults will set and enforce clear limits and boundaries. They will be consistent in enforcing these, and remain regulated when holding limits.

The emphasis here is Stand 2, where parents are guided to focus their energy and enthusiasm on their children when things are going well. It invites parents to applaud and commend children for any accomplishment—even tiny ones.

A useful format is to say, "I see you _____," or "I notice _____," or "You are . . . " For example:

"I see you patting the dog gently."
"You got your shirt into the laundry hamper."
"I notice you tasted your green beans."
"You are working on math problem number five."
"I see you came to the table for dinner right on time!"
"You are already putting your homework in your bookbag for tomorrow."

As parents carefully and mindfully observe children, they will come to notice how many opportunities there are to acknowledge what's going right. Noticing what's going right includes noticing what isn't going wrong. If a child is having trouble with hitting, for example, parents can make a point of mentioning that they notice that the child is not hitting. This may seem silly to parents at first, but it is nourishing to comment, "It's dinnertime and you haven't hit all day. You are very kind!" Or "Even though your sister took your toy, you just yelled—you didn't hit at all! I see you working hard to manage your anger."

Parents can be taught not to let an hour go by without appreciating and pointing out things that are going well, as well as the absence of any behavior they are eager to get rid of. The point of these observations is to bring children's attention to anything they are doing that is good, acceptable, or not causing problems, and to help them feel seen and appreciated in those moments. They begin to receive repeated messages that they are on track and being successful in this moment.

To take a shower
The child must . . .

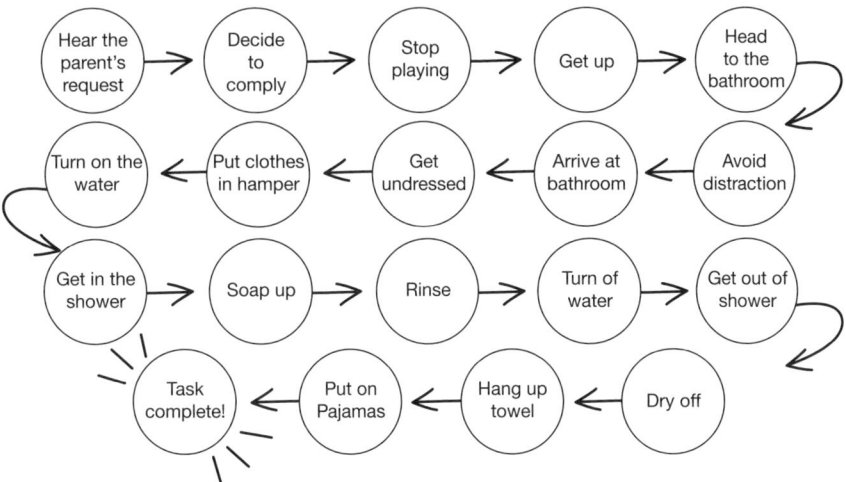

Figure 14.1 Steps to Take a Shower SOURCE: © Eva Kornerup

Recognitions like these also exercise attunement in the moment, which is an essential component of a secure relationship. Parents pay close attention to their children and mirror what they are doing and feeling. They don't wait for full-blown success as they may have previously defined it, but acknowledge and praise small steps toward excellence.

This approach is powerful in fostering children's cooperation—and good for therapists to know, as defiance is a common presenting concern in psychotherapy. Making an effort to notice positive trends is important because much of what parents expect of children requires extended focus and follow-through, even if the adults don't think of it that way. For instance, to complete the task of taking a shower, a child must complete a long series of steps, with each presenting new opportunities for distraction (Figure 14.1).

Completion of any one of these steps can be recognized as a victory on the path to success. Rather than waiting for the process to be completed before offering praise, productive parents can see their opening at any (or several) of these points:

"I see you stopped playing and are getting ready to head to the bathroom."
"You are turning on the water—you're taking care of business!"
"I notice you are drying off already!"

Each of these comments creates momentum to drive children to move on through the steps of getting the task done. Interacting positively and enthusiastically when children are doing well takes advantage of teachable moments.

TARGETED STRATEGIES FOR RECOGNITION

To support adults in transforming their relationship with children in their care, NHA provides a detailed breakdown of strategies for positive recognition.

Active recognition. Purposefully notice and articulate when good or neutral behavior is happening.

"You are brushing your hair."
"I see you watching cartoons and laughing."
"I notice you remembered to take out the trash."

Experiential recognition. Purposefully notice and articulate when values are being demonstrated.

"You are a hard worker; you already finished your math. That shows such dedication to your studies."
"I see you putting away your clean laundry. That shows your responsibility and helpfulness."

Proactive recognition. Purposefully notice and articulate when misbehavior is absent.

"It is 9 a.m. already, and you haven't yelled all morning."

"You could have been rude to me when I forgot to give you money for your field trip, but instead, you just reminded me kindly."

Creative recognition. Purposefully notice and articulate when the child's behavior is trending in the right direction.

"David, time for your homework. I see you already heading toward your backpack."
"I notice you've already started picking up your laundry off the floor."
"I need you to empty the dishwasher; there you go, you're already starting."

Recommend to parents that they provide recognitions at least once an hour. Twice an hour is even more powerful. These comments should be felt with the heart, articulated with detail, and delivered with sincerity and enthusiasm.

REINFORCING POSITIVE TRENDS: FEEDING OPPOSITES

The key to helping parents combat misbehavior is teaching them to take a positive perspective. Even highly aggressive children are not hitting every minute of every day. We recommend having parents comment at any nonhitting moment, even if hitting just occurred five minutes earlier: "I notice you are not hitting now; you are showing excellent self-control and respect for your sister." This is a way of getting a foot in the door toward building the skill of not hitting.

Whenever parents notice any behavior or attitude they don't want, advise them to use restraint and have them begin hunting for examples of that problem not occurring. Help them to focus on the absence of the problem.

- Is the child's irresponsibility annoying? Have them focus on responsibility when children have just shown an example of it: "I see you let the dog outside without a reminder. Well done! Your responsibility shows you care for him."
- Are they tired of messes? Have them notice even the smallest sign of

attention to neatness: "Thank you for putting your dish in the sink, Carol. You are very neat and considerate." This approach is a way to teach neatness while instilling positive self-image.

- Is rudeness the issue? Have the parent focus on courteous responses: "You just said you don't want to go in a polite tone and without cursing; that makes it easy for me to listen to your reasons. I appreciate your courtesy."

This style of parenting is highly sensitive to nuance. Rather than waiting for a clear example of good behavior, parents attend to any hint of good conduct. Any sign of the ultimate goal of kindness, gentleness, self-control, or cooperation is worthy of recognition. Parents have the privilege of giving warmth to any trace of a virtue they wish to encourage.

Initially, as parents begin to use this style of teaching, it may feel odd to them and their children. Encourage them to persist; it is worth the effort. The positive attunement inherent in this process feels safe to children and fosters secure attachment. Attending to successes, rather than failures, creates a trusting connection and bolsters children's self-confidence. Over time, positive recognition comes to set the tone of the relationship; this, in turn, builds trust and encourages positive behaviors. Significant decreases in inattention and decreased impulsivity and hyperactivity have been documented using this approach (see Nuño et al., 2020).

Children may reject recognitions that feel insincere or like an attempt to manipulate them. Most children sense when a comment is misattuned. Sincere recognitions require that parents reflect on what is right at this moment. What is important? What valuable traits are children manifesting right now? Help parents dig deep, tune in to their love for their children, and identify: What about this moment is terrific? What about their children is amazing? When experiencing these sincere feelings of appreciation, most parents can find deeply nourishing acknowledgments that not only shift children's behavior but also nourish their souls. Note that the feelings of joy and connection created by these comments calm the nervous system and release oxytocin, the hormone associated with peace and contentment.

Recognition of success is positive teaching. Rule of thumb: Where parents pay attention to behaviors, children will engage in those behaviors more often. As children note what is appreciated and recognized, they do more of that. Each time they hear a compliment about their behavior that feels true, they file it away as a success. Each positive comment serves as fertilizer to grow the action it addresses and encourages the repetition of that behavior (Nuño et al., 2020). This is how we feed opposites—by seeking out the opposite of the problematic behavior and fueling that.

EXAMPLE: TEENS RECOGNIZE A TEACHABLE MOMENT

As high school seniors, my son Joshua and his friend Jacob worked as cotechnical directors on a play. Their job included supervising the strike—closing down and cleaning up when the show finished. They found this a most challenging job. Some of the cast members were not interested in laboring to tear down the set, stow the props and costumes, sweep, and organize. A few students literally hid elsewhere in the theater to avoid being assigned a job.

Jacob and Joshua chose not to confront their fellow students at the time. They discussed the problem and decided against verbal confrontation, recognizing that any direct criticism would lead to an argument. Joshua said, "Let's do this thing my mom and dad do . . . call people out for doing a good job instead of calling them out for doing a bad job."

They decided to create a post on Facebook that would be visible to the entire cast and crew. The post thanked them for their hard work during the production of the show and the strike and specifically named those who worked hard. They chose not to name anyone who neglected work. The boys said it was a "cathartic experience" for them because they felt they "handled it appropriately and responsibly. Also, the people who worked well took note and continued to work well. They felt validated."

E. S.

CLEAR, CHILD-FRIENDLY RULES

Although many households run without the benefit of well-articulated rules, explicitly stating rules supports clarity about the expectations at home for both parents and children. This clarity adds security and predictability to children's lives. Clarity of expectations is especially crucial for intense or persistent children. Children and parents need to know what is expected, what is in bounds, and what is out of bounds, with no confusing gray areas. To facilitate this process, therapists can encourage parents to create a set of house rules that are very specific and child friendly. Child-friendly rules are, believe it or not, negatively worded to add clarity.

Consider the often-used rule, "Be respectful." How easy is it to tell whether this rule is being followed? If you stop and consider your day today, were you respectful when driving? With your spouse and children? At the store? It's probably unclear. If you are like most people, you can come up with moments in the day when you question whether your actions were respectful. "Hmm . . . I did come to a rolling stop at that corner. I did not greet the cashier when she said hello. Maybe I've been underperforming in the area of respect."

Now, consider the negatively worded rule "No cursing." Think about your day again; have you been cursing? Much clearer. It is easy to tell whether you've followed this rule or not. For this reason, clear, child-friendly rules are prohibitive rules: no arguing; no whining; no aggression.

When working with parents, we advise creating household rules together in session. Parents can be encouraged to post rules where they can see them and be reminded of them, but rules do not need to be unveiled in a family meeting or posted for kids to see. What leads children to focus on rules more intently and to make a more considerable effort to follow them is not a conversation or a poster, but rather the positive feedback they receive when following them.

Once household rules are complete, remind parents: Positivity reigns supreme. Children are more open to learning when they are feeling successful and happy. The emphasis is not on catching children breaking the rules, but on catching them following the rules. Rules are taught most effectively by celebrating when children comply with them. Parents must stop and say out loud that they see their children following the rules.

Parents can add to their flow of specific, positive recognitions that cover rule following:

> "I noticed you have not whined all morning. Good job following that rule!"
>
> "Your sister took your toy, and you told me right away instead of hitting. Well done!" (Even if the child was yelling, at least he didn't break the no hitting rule.)

Therapists can remind parents that the goal is to help children's brains connect the good feeling of being recognized and appreciated with their ability to self-control—an illustration of Hebb's rule, "Neurons that fire together wire together."

A Few Details on Rules

The key to successful rules is specificity. If parents need the rule "No wiping boogers on the counter," then they should add it. Children benefit from this level of clarity. If that means having lots of rules, that is okay—this ultimately provides more opportunities for positive recognition. If a new rule is required, it is fine to add it at the moment. No need to wait. Parents can just announce, "New rule! No throwing food at the table."

Therapists should keep in mind that not all families need the same rules. Parents' creation of rules should take into account their family's culture and values and their children's specific needs. For example, some families may need the rule "No talking in church." Others may need clarity around "No breaking the law," while others absolutely cannot get by without the rule "No iPad in the bathtub."

Remember, parents' focus remains on moments when rules are followed. This is consistent with the core principles: Stand 1—Absolutely No, and Stand 2—Absolutely Yes. Parental energetic focus and passion are no longer imparted for children's misbehavior. Misbehavior is met with a low-key response. Rule-following behavior is met with high responsiveness and authentic enthusiasm.

RESPONDING TO MISBEHAVIOR MINDFULLY

After parents create clear, child-friendly rules, and commit to not over-reacting to broken rules and hunting for examples of children following the rules, the foundation is set for dealing with misbehavior—for enacting Stand 3 clarity. By now, with all the focus on the positives, parents are probably wondering what to do when children are misbehaving. At these times, therapists can recommend they actually do very little.

This approach does not imply that parents never correct misbehavior, but rather that they correct mindfully, mildly, without anger, hostility, belittling, disdain, debates, or quarrels. Correction should be done without investing passion because a corrective moment is not a learning moment. Parents may need support to learn not to attempt discussion when they are upset, or when children are upset. The intervention is, "No hitting, Tommy." And then, "Thank you for stopping hitting."

Adults may feel drawn to explain their position, chastise, scold, or lecture children, but should avoid this at all costs. The time to discuss the importance of self-control is when children are exhibiting self-control, not when they are not. When parents are calm and not lecturing, speaking loudly, or threatening, they avoid activating children's defensive brains. As a result, defiance, tears, or tantrums are less likely to arise.

If children insist on engaging when energy is high, it is useful for parents to repeat the limits with a calm voice, using the "broken record" technique. This method consists of not explaining or letting children lead the interaction astray with arguing; instead, merely hold the limit.

"You may not hit."

"But he hit me first! You always pick on me. I only touched him. . . . "

"Nonetheless, you may not hit."

This less energetic response limits parents' escalation and (often) children's escalation too. Therapists can remind parents that even this style of calm and mild correction, while necessary, is not the moment of most powerful learning; it is not a teachable moment. The aim is to move past it and into Stand 2 recognition, where true learning can happen.

CLASSIC TIME-OUT:
A CONSEQUENCE FOR MISBEHAVIOR

Time-out is a common approach often attempted to change children's behavior. The classic understanding of time-out as a behavioral intervention is described here. Later, we will lay out a modified version of time-out called reset, which is more relationally sensitive and attachment-sound.

Correctly applied, time-out is not a punishment, but rather the absence of all rewards. Check Table 14.1, which will probably remind you of your Psychology 101 undergraduate course. It explains *operant conditioning*, the use of rewards and punishments to alter behavior. As you can see, there are four ways to use a positive or negative consequence to change behavior with a reward or punishment. As used in the laboratory, one can either add or remove a reward or a punishment to change behavior.

Table 14.1 OPERANT CONDITIONING		
	Add	**Remove**
Reward	1. Positive reinforcement (reward) • Give praise/attention • Create fun/play • Give toy • Give treat Example: Giving candy to a child for taking a bath increases child's willingness to take a bath.	2. Negative punishment (absence of reward) • Cease praise/attention • Cease fun/play • Remove toy • Remove treat Example: Taking away candy for hitting decreases child's hitting.
Punishment	3. Positive punishment • Give extra chores • Write _____100 times • Spanking Example: Giving an extra chore for hitting decreases child's hitting.	4. Negative reinforcement • Free pass from chores • Excused from homework Example: Relieving a child of his chore for taking a bath increases child's willingness to take a bath.

Therapists will recognize that typical parenting practices use all four types of behavioral consequences. For example, parents are practicing operant conditioning when they use recognitions with their children; each positive comment is a deposit of attention and warmth in response to their behavior. This practice is a reward, which serves to increase the frequency of that behavior. The other boxes of this chart are also used in popular parenting; for example, when a parent spanks a child, they are adding a punishment to decrease the preceding behavior. When parents remove a punishment—giving a free pass from chores in response to a child's good behavior, for example—they are attempting to increase the frequency of that behavior.

For a reward or a punishment to be effective, it must be powerful. A weak reward is not effective in changing behavior. If parents attempt to use a sticker to influence children's behavior, they will usually find it fruitless and may suspect they need to find a stronger reward. A punishment also needs to be powerful enough to make an impact. A stern look or a raised voice is not sufficiently strong to make an impact on many children. Of course, these children might respond to harsher punishment; but while it may change their behavior, harsh punishment has very destructive effects on children and the parent–child relationship.

In addition to these drawbacks of punishment, therapists should also keep in mind—and remind parents—that actions thought of as punishment may not feel like punishment to some children. While interventions like yelling, scolding, and lecturing are highly upsetting and stressful to some children, others experience them as intense moments of connection with parents: a rich reward of attention and energy. When parents are lecturing, children are the undisputed focus of their parents' attention and passion. Many children are confused by the simultaneous pleasure of being the sole recipient of the parent's attention and distress at the negativity of the attention.

Box 2, the absence of reward, is the cell that best represents the practice of time-out. Time-out is not intended to be a punishment. It is meant to discourage unwanted behavior by removing anything that might reward the behavior. Over time, typical use of time-out has shifted it away from the intent of no reward to a view that it is a punishment. It is inappropriately implemented after threats, includes shame-provoking actions, and tends to be overly long and isolating. It is due to this shift away from the research-validated application of time-out that this intervention often fails and is falling out of favor.

Problems With the Use of Time-Out in Real Life

As time-out has moved out of the laboratory and into general use by parents and teachers, it has drifted from its theoretical origins in operant conditioning into various new forms. Some drawbacks of this transition are the addition of various tasks to increase children's aversion to it—a misguided attempt to use negativity to teach. Parents may require a child to think about what they have done; to list better choices they could make next time; to write an apology; or to stay in the time-out chair for one minute per year of age (we are not sure where that came from).

While these versions of time-out are not cruel, they are not consistent with time-out as a simple removal of rewards. They are also difficult to implement without giving children a level of engagement and focus that may inadvertently turn time-out into a game, a new stressor, or a new reward. Additionally, lengthy time-outs tend to create anger, resentment, and refusal to comply, which is not useful and overly energizes the negative interaction.

A second problem with time-out as it is often practiced is the inclusion of isolation and dismissal as part of its implementation. Therapists can remind parents that when children are upset or misbehaving, they almost always have a reason. Sending children to their room, making them sit alone, or otherwise giving them the cold shoulder does not communicate support or understanding. Misbehaving children often need help to regulate—think coregulation—and cutting them off from support does not help. Such harshly applied, isolating time-outs are painful to children and do not move families toward the ultimate goal of creating a stable, loving, supportive relationship that can sustain children as they grow.

RESET: THE NURTURED HEART
APPROACH TO CONSEQUENCE

The implementation of time-out prescribed by NHA is called *reset*. It is a pause in the continuous flow of recognition and appreciation the parents give to their children. Scrupulously applied resets are a way of ensuring children are not inadvertently rewarded for misbehavior while simultaneously serving the purpose of signaling "no" to the preceding behavior.

Reset occurs wherever the family is; there is no need for a unique time-out chair or place. There are no threats or warnings; if misbehavior occurs, parents merely say, "reset," wait until the behavior ceases, and then warmly say, "Thank you for resetting." It is that simple. Children should not be asked to think about or do anything while resetting. However, while the child is in reset, it is critical that parents remain calm. No lecturing, glaring at, or grabbing children; parental body language and eye contact remain soft. The tone set during reset should be one of patient neutrality. Since, by this point, parents have already created a steady flow of recognition for success, the absence of enthusiastic attention and recognition is the key to reset. It feels dull and unexciting to children. After many repetitions children will eventually conclude, "I don't want another reset. . . . They're no fun." The parental attitude of neutrality avoids the stress and tension of more harsh consequences and allows children to see parents as a safe harbor and calm presence in times of upset and a resource when help is needed. A proper reset is untimed and very brief; it is over when the misbehavior ends.

After the reset, parents immediately focus attention and commentary on anything positive that preceded the error, such as efforts to self-control; or that followed it, such as apologies, leaving the area, or efforts to self-calm. Returning to Stand 2, parents resume the flow of positives and recognition without holding a grudge or harping on the child's error. The misbehavior is left in the past and all parental energy returns to seeing and recognizing success: "Good job with that reset." More challenging children may resist the reset and work to undermine it, but if parents remain consistent and calm, those children eventually realize that the reset is no big deal. Most will come around to complying and getting it over with.

Parents may feel discouraged if initially, the child does not stop the misbehavior quickly, or if they stop and then immediately restart. At these times, parents merely reset the child again, keeping their energy very low, and remain prepared to quickly and enthusiastically recognize the behaviors stopping whenever they do end. A word of caution: Reset is not effective in the absence of a rich connection (time-in). If parents are using the reset but slacking off on frequent, rich recognitions, reset will fail.

Therapists can help parents to prepare for some predictable challenges in implementing the reset. For example, a child might refuse to reset. They may attempt to argue. They may ignore their parents altogether. This behavior can create a predicament for parents, who may feel tempted to escalate. But there is no need to respond to any attempts to dodge the reset. The child's behavior will subside eventually. Even if it takes a long time for this to happen, parental escalation is not helpful, either from a relational perspective or for the purpose of calming the interaction. You can remind parents that they are removing the rewards of their passionate attention, so that means removing threats, lectures, grimaces, sneers, sighs of exasperation, and harsh eye contact.

Properly used, the reset is brief and demands minimal parental attention and energy. It is essentially a short period in which children receive nothing enjoyable or intense, yet they are supported in their own calming by the presence of calm adults. Resets are not just for times of major rule infractions; they should be used every time a rule is broken, the first time the rule is broken, with no warnings, reminders, or second chances.

PARENTS TEACHING RESET

Resets are not only for children. Parents can reset themselves frequently. When they catch themselves doing something that runs counter to their sense of what's appropriate and right—speeding, raising their voice at their spouse, on the verge of snapping at a clerk—and choose to stop and get back on a positive track, they have reset.

Aggressive and disrespectful impulses are part of our human nature. Mature, adaptive people have frequent experiences of self-restraint. Parents' relationships with their children benefit when they are not too proud to reset themselves in interaction with children. Doing so overtly and out loud is a way of teaching children by example how and when to reset.

Parents can model the reset for their children by saying, "I'm sorry I raised my voice; I'm going to reset myself now." They can pause briefly, get back on track, and resume their interaction. If they are agitated, they can actually say they need to reset, leave the area, calm down, and then return. By doing this overtly, parents teach their children that there is no shame in changing one's behavior or in taking the time they need to restrain their impulses. The learning is both explicit and implicit.

Inherently, children feel angry or humiliated when told to stop doing something. Being told by parents to reset is no different. But when parents model the reset by resetting themselves, they teach that all people have reason to reset sometimes, and that it is no cause for embarrassment or chagrin. The real lesson to children is there is no shame in stopping oneself when on a path to nowhere good, and that this is something all people must practice.

Therapists can follow these steps to help parents teach reset to their families:

1. Modeling the reset. Have parents begin by demonstrating the reset out loud and in front of children. Let children see parents reset themselves frequently. Children learn by observation as they repeatedly hear their parents announce that they are going to reset, then see them pause, breathe, and reengage calmly.

2. Recognizing children's spontaneous resets. After modeling the reset themselves for a few weeks, parents can move on to recognizing children's spontaneous resets, praising them when they have calmed themselves of their own accord. For example, when an angry child storms off to his room, slams the door, and emerges calmly 15 minutes later, the parents can praise the child with an authentic smile and say, "Excellent reset; you calmed yourself down with no help at all. You have awesome self-awareness and self-control."

3. Resetting self and child at the same time. The next step is for parents to reset themselves and their children at the same time. "Yikes, we watched

that show for a full hour. Let's reset and get back to chores," or "This conversation is escalating; let's reset and talk about this again later."

4. Resetting the child. Then, finally, parents can begin to reset their children. A simple calmly stated "reset" after misbehavior is all it takes. Have them wait until the behavior halts and then immediately, with authenticity, recognize children for resetting. If the problem behavior does not stop, or if it escalates, parents reset the behavior again, being ready to energize the slightest move in the right direction.

POST-RESET: MAKING AMENDS AND BACKGROUND CONSEQUENCES

Within the context of this parenting approach, additional consequences can be applied occasionally and judiciously. This may be called for in two circumstances: (1) where making amends is useful, and (2) where children break a significant rule repeatedly without the ability to reset in a reasonable amount of time, usually because the rule breaking is very gratifying.

Making amends or providing a service to the offended person can offer children a sense of closure and repair. We suggest using this strategy only when children's reset (meaning stopping the behavior) is not enough. For example, cursing requires no consequence beyond reset. If children reset and stop the cursing, it is over, and parents can return to time-in, which is time in connection—time with the adult that is fun, intimate, warm, and relational. Hitting, however, is a different story. If a child hurts another person, it is helpful to the relationship that the child helps the hurt person. These reparations are suggested, never forced, after the fact, and only when everyone involved is calm again. Reparations might be doing a chore for the person who was hurt or giving a gift of a treat or toy. The child who broke the rules can decide, when things are calm, how to make amends. And amends are done in a state of time-in. During amends, adults are engaged, cheerful, and helpful, recognizing the child for their effort.

Another example is when property is destroyed. Let's say a child breaks a door while in the throes of a tantrum. The parent resets himself. He resets the child. When the child eventually calms down, the reset is praised. Later, when everyone is peaceful, the parent and child can go to the hardware store, get what is needed to fix the door, and do it together. The door fixing is done in a state of time-in, with positive connection, recognitions, and laughter. Parents do this without holding a grudge or revisiting the offense. Of course, the child may refuse, but typically if there is no shaming and the interaction around fixing the door is pleasant, most children will go right along. Over time these kinds of repairs become part of the fabric of life, unremarkable and natural.

Another type of intervention that may accompany reset is the use of what we call *background consequences*. Background consequences never take center stage, but are part of the understood structure of the home. One example is when parents are struggling to get screen time under control. They set a clear rule that the next day's screen time is contingent on turning the iPad off when told. If the child dawdles, he loses tomorrow's screen time. The child is informed of this ahead of time, at a time when everyone is calm. The next time he dawdles, he is not reminded or threatened with the loss; he is just told to reset. The next day the screen time is not available, and the consequence is applied without lecture or admonition. While the child is not allowed to use screens, the adults hold no grudge; life goes on as usual with fun, pleasant interactions and recognition for successes.

Avoiding Harshness

Even these low-key, matter-of-fact consequences can open the door to harsh and punitive interactions for some families. The addition of consequences can be a slippery slope. It is common and natural for parents to want to do something big to get their children's attention and to increase motivation to behave well. Endorsing any consequence can cause a cascade into this habit of launching bigger and bigger punishments to try to get the child to stop breaking rules. Within our recommended parenting approach, consequences are used very rarely. We suggest only one target behavior have a background consequence in place at a time, and that a new one is only added when the prior one is mastered and the consequence is no longer needed. Background consequences are always created ahead of time when all are calm, are communicated to the child ahead of time when misbehavior is not occurring, and are never created in the heat of the moment.

When working with parents, keep an eye out for the reemergence of punitive practices and overuse of consequences. We have often observed backsliding into fewer and fewer recognitions and overreliance on negativity when consequences are endorsed. The most powerful principles of this parenting approach remain regular use of positive recognitions, withholding extra energy when misbehavior occurs, clarity in rules and expectations, and parents resetting themselves and their children. Consequences are always of secondary importance and can be done away with altogether. The real intervention is the regularly offered recognition, which helps children feel seen, appreciated, and on track, and serves to energize them to escalate their efforts to do what is appreciated, again and again.

THE ENERGY OF RESET

The key to an effective reset is the parents' physical and emotional state. Relational energy—the level of adult passion and connection in relationship to children—is the subtext of the interaction that makes the reset helpful or condemns it to fail.

As we have discussed, many children, especially emotionally intense children, are attracted to interpersonal energy, often even negative energy. These children will go for the bigger energetic experience every time. Anxious or traumatized children, on the other hand, are often avoidant of intense energy. They react with panic, flares of anger, or loss of control when relational energy is too intense or is negative. They often respond poorly to the intense energy that some parents release in the face of problems or misbehavior. Neither type of child learns well when discipline is laden with negativity.

Reset, therefore, must be used with the lowest possible emission of energy. Resetting with low energy can be hard and is an acquired skill—especially in light of the fact that moments when parents choose to reset children for breaking rules are also moments where parental agitation is often high or mounting. This makes it challenging to keep the energy of the interaction low. Parents who are skillful at keeping their emotional expressiveness muted during reset are more effective.

Teach parents that relational energy is expressed and experienced both verbally and nonverbally and is picked up by both the left brain and right brain. Most parents are highly aware of sending and receiving verbal messages from others and understand that speech carries within it a message of attention, interest, and relationship. But the subtleties of nonverbal communication are often overlooked. Humans of all ages are observant of gaze, body language, posture, tone of voice, facial expression, the pace of interaction, and touch as means of relational connection (Siegel, 2015). The right brain perceives these means of communication. When this nonverbal communication is intense or passionate during reset, it sends powerful energy that can contradict the intended message and undermine the success of this disciplinary strategy.

Energy Leaks

Both verbal and nonverbal communication can occur at mild or intense levels. It is relatively simple to notice expressions of negative energy like yelling, lecturing, grabbing, or indulging in disdainful talk. More subtle deviations from the low-energy path can be difficult to discern. These small leaks of negative energy can nevertheless have a strong influence on an interaction. Common leaks include:

- A sour look
- A heavy sigh
- A reminder of the rules
- A focus on children's noncompliance
- Escalating consequences out of annoyance
- A tone of impatience or sarcasm
- Hard looks or stare-downs
- Not enforcing a rule or giving a second chance
- Engaging in a detailed discussion of children's mistakes
- Scowling

- Eye rolling
- Throwing up hands

Therapists can help parents to recognize that each of these leaks is a slip away from the intention to energize only children's excellent traits and to refuse to make their passion and connection available for misbehavior. Of course, children will notice if they get more of their parents' time and attention through misconduct than through positive behavior.

Even small leaks will undercut parents' desire to foster their children's wonderful traits. If parents can identify these slips, they can stay aware and stop leaks in their tracks. They can reset themselves to embody their overarching principle of energizing what is wonderful in themselves and their children.

PARENT EMOTIONAL REGULATION: TEACHING PARENTS TO RESET

Let's face it: Parenting is hard! It is especially hard to remain calm when children are struggling. But it is critical to the functioning of this system that parents build their capacity to maintain self-control, even when it is hard. To this end, we recommend spending the necessary time to help parents take ownership of their own reset.

Learning to regulate one's own intense emotions is an integral aspect of being a successful parent and a prerequisite to teaching children to regulate themselves. Therapists can facilitate parents resetting themselves by discussing explicitly that they must learn to reset and to calm themselves to stay on track and adhere to their parenting ideals. A good starting point is to discuss the triggers and the emotions that result when triggered and to clarify the behaviors they want to demonstrate when parenting is challenging. This is also linked closely to parents fostering their own access to a mindful state. As described earlier in this book, there are many ways to build mindfulness, and parents who practice mindfulness build their ability to reset (think regulate) when it is hard.

This initial exploration is more like adult psychotherapy, with the caveats that it is in service of the children and does not go as deep or last as long as individual psychotherapy. Once parents have greater clarity on their intended responses to challenging family moments, you can introduce specific ways to reset.

When parenting is difficult, parents can learn to mindfully notice what they feel in their body. Some signs that they are not doing well may include a pounding heart, pressure in the head, tension in the throat, or a sense of urgency. Parents can also pause in difficult moments to notice their thoughts, which may include confusion, racing or pressured thoughts, or highly negative ideas about themselves or their children. They may notice an intense urge to engage negatively to make their point or to make unwanted behaviors stop. Once parents recognize they are feeling angry, agitated, or out of control, they can use self-soothing skills to calm themselves. Instead of letting their passion carry them away, they can step back, reset, and work to reconnect with their calmer selves (Naumburg, 2019).

There is no right or wrong length of time for parents or children to take as a reset. A reset can occur in an instant—a deep breath, a quick thought of "I'm committed to not spanking," and jumping back on track. Some resets take longer and may require parents to take more of a break. They may need to walk away, wash their face, lie down for a bit, and then reengage. Sometimes an even more extended break is needed: a shower, time listening to music, or a talk with a friend before they regain their composure. There is no correct length of time for a reset. For parents resetting themselves, they can consider it over when they feel reset.

As is the case with any long-term personal goal (think school, exercise, budgets), successful parenting is achieved because people do not give up when they slip up. Therapists can help parents preemptively create their own reset options, a self-care list, and an emergency recovery list for use in tough parenting moments. Some common reset and self-care examples are deep breathing, counting to 10, or focusing on a productive thought such as "I will not be derailed; this is important" or "I'm going to go ahead and do what works instead of what feels good." Some parents find that it is helpful to take five deep breaths, internally recite a mantra, or leave the room until they are calm. Others find taking the time to engage large muscle groups by walking, running, or stretching can be calming. This list is highly personal and must be created and endorsed by the parents themselves to be useful.

PRACTICE AND MODEL RESET IN THERAPY

To create positive experiences with reset, work with clients to cultivate the understanding that it is healthy and honorable to reset. Demonstrate that therapists can reset too by modeling resetting during sessions. We suggest this be done freely and cheerfully. As therapists, we automatically reset ourselves when we interrupt, distract a client, or behave impulsively, and it is useful to do this out loud with clients. We also reset back to the topic when a conversation shifts to chitchat or superficial discussion.

Experienced and confident therapists can reset clients when their work is not productive. A client in an extended rant or self-deprecating monologue can be reset by the therapist. Resetting an adult requires the relationship to be well established and secure for the client. Reset must be an act of love and a demonstration that the therapist wants only the best for the client. Saying the word "reset" out loud at these times serves to set a limit in the most loving, accepting, and calm of ways.

The ultimate goal is to help parents understand that the reset provides an emotional and behavioral pause—a way to shift from a negative or ineffective path to resume acting out of hope and goodness. Resetting is making an about-face away from adversity, yelling, or withdrawing and back to a calm, integrated, and centered self that is available for healthy connection. An adult reset is another form of reflective practice: As parents pay attention to the process of calming and accepting the situation, they learn what works best to get themselves back on track toward their overarching goals.

YOUR PRACTICE AND THE NURTURED HEART APPROACH: IN SUMMARY

We hope that you will find, as we have, that NHA is a powerful and accessible way for parents to quickly shift negative dynamics in a positive direction. The approach offers particular advantages for children in that calm and energetically aware parents can recognize and connect with them even when children are overwhelmed (or overwhelming). When parents confidently settle into the realization that they have a playbook for parenting, they feel freer to see that their children's behaviors are expressing their underlying needs. Awareness of the energetic components of parenting helps parents correct children's behavior without dismissing their underlying needs and feelings. A low-energy response to misbehavior does not forego parental curiosity about its origins or parental support and kindness toward children's felt needs.

Once this system of parenting is in place, parents have created optimal conditions for learning to occur, and children can be free to learn from their mistakes. At this juncture, parents accept that misbehavior will happen and respond to it with low energy. This is how children, who are experiential learners, learn parameters. In a positive and safe home environment, they are free to try different things. Typically children will try behaviors parents are delighted to see and behaviors they hope never to see again, and discover what each produces for them in the world.

It is not parents' job to prevent misbehavior, but rather to allow misbehavior to lead to learning. We want parents' responses to simply give information to children, such as, "Disruptive behavior does not bring good things," or "This behavior is embraced."

A FOUNDATION FOR REGULATION: PARENTAL MINDFULNESS AND SELF-CARE

Interestingly, while reset occurs in the moment of dysregulation, the ability to reset has its roots in actions and patterns that occur far in advance of the stressful moment. Beyond teaching parents to rest themselves while in stressful situations, it is beneficial to also encourage parents to strengthen their base emotional resources. This process begins by developing self-awareness and prioritizing self-care. When parents neglect their own physical and mental health, they are more vulnerable to impulsive, emotion-driven parenting choices. When parents establish mindful habits that stabilize their bodies and minds, they can respond more thoughtfully in the moment and more quickly return to calm and stability when things are chaotic or heated. Remember that the key is practice. We get better at anything with rehearsal. Neurons that fire together wire together.

As presented earlier, parents do their best parenting when they are emotionally and mentally stable, using their higher mental capacity to make decisions. At these times, they are flexible in their thinking and behavior; they can observe how their children are receiving their actions and adjust accordingly. They can adjust their speech, tone, and body language to communicate with their children calmly and lovingly. Even if they are telling children to stop a behavior or giving a consequence, they can do so with respect and dignity. They are using their higher mind to regulate themselves, moderate their intensity, and support their efforts to do what works instead of what feels good in the moment.

The norms for our society include any number of habits and cultural mores that contribute to adults' likelihood of dysregulation. It is common for adults to miss out on sleep, eat poorly or irregularly, and lack exercise and healthy movement in their lives. Our nervous systems are barraged by excessive busyness, lack of alone time, noise, multitasking, and rushing. The amount of time we spend with our devices is extensive and ever-expanding. There is growing evidence that interfacing with screens overstimulates and stresses our brains, which makes us more edgy. Many overwhelmed parents lack social support and others to turn to for help and to normalize parenting strains (Naumburg, 2019). With the addition of high-stress family circumstances such as mental illness, excessive family conflict, or the loss of a family member, a parent wellness plan is crucial. This plan can make the difference between a positive process through conflict or a downward spiral of negativity.

Therapists can help parents monitor the level of overall family stress, which affects the whole system. Parents can learn to pay attention to the pacing of the family's activities, the frequency with which they pause for relaxing time together, and how often they take time for play or for being with nurturing family friends. Parents can improve their self-regulation skills through a myriad of mindfulness practices, as discussed earlier: journaling, mindful meditation, yoga, prayer, or other reflective and soothing activities (see Part III).

In some cases, parents may bring in deeper personal issues that stand in the way of their developing habits conducive to good self-regulation such as a history of trauma, recent grief, addiction, or unhealthy relationship patterns. In this case, the therapist might choose to work with parents on a more intimate level or may decide to refer parents to an individual therapist. Either way, the development of a parent's emotional health and resources will increase calm in the family and minimize emotional distress and conflict (Fosha et al., 2009). Parents are the heart of the family, and their mental health sets parameters for the family's emotional health.

Learning to regulate one's own intense feelings is a critical part of being a successful parent and a prerequisite to teaching children to soothe themselves. Knowing when and how to calm oneself helps set the tone when children need help with soothing. Allan Schore (2012) notes, "In order to act as a regulator of the infant's arousal, the mother (parent) must be able to regulate her own arousal state" (p. 229). When parents find themselves emotionally dysregulated, it is their job to slow down, resist impulses, self-correct, and take time to calm and reconnect with their prefrontal cortex before taking action. They can also ask for emotional support from friends, family, or a therapist to reach a state of calm and transition back to emotional stability. Only then can they move forward with steady kindness.

REPAIR AFTER PARENT–CHILD DISCONNECTION

> Understanding alone cannot prevent disrupted connections from occurring. Some will inevitably happen. The challenge we all share is to embrace our humanity with humor and patience so that we can in turn relate to our children with openness and kindness. To continually chastise ourselves for our "errors" with our children keeps us involved in our own emotional issues and out of relationship with our children.
>
> DANIEL J. SIEGEL AND MARY HARTZELL,
> *PARENTING FROM THE INSIDE-OUT*

Family therapists can keep in mind that conflict between parents and children is inevitable. Even the most thoughtfully applied limits and consequences can leave family members with hurt feelings. Parents can accomplish limit setting using our suggested approaches without excess negativity, but uncomfortable feelings may still arise. At these times, when children naturally dislike the application of consequences, or parents have lost their cool, a break occurs in the flow of positive regard and support. This rupture may require repair.

If parents have lost their temper or released negative energy on their children with harsh words or action, it is beneficial for the therapist to coach them to make repairs and attend to reestablishing harmony, connection, and understanding. After children introduce negativity with aggression, defiance, or other acting out, this is also a time for repair.

Relational repair is typically needed when children or parents are hurt, holding a grudge, or feeling alienated, rejected, or disconnected from each other. The time to repair is any time there has been a rupture in the flow of positive connection that parents are striving for, whether the misstep was the parents' or the children's fault. Responsibility always rests with parents to reset their own emotions or address children's hurt feelings, and to repair if needed to create or restore parental attunement and stable attachment presence.

If parents ask why they should seek to repair with their children when they are not the only ones responsible for the rupture, remind them that building up negativity and distance can lead to ongoing alienation, hurt, resentment, and even revenge. If these feelings are not addressed, they can damage children's sense of safety and trust, which can harm the attachment relationship. Such feelings also hurt children's self-image, as they can cause children to incorporate a view of themselves as unloved, bad, or damaged. Finally, unprocessed feelings prevent children from learning about painful emotions and resolving conflict. Instead, parents should take initiative to shift relationship dynamics to a repair mode, to restart the flow of understanding, support, and appreciation.

It is important to note that children often feel shame and insecurity after their own mistakes. While awareness of their mistakes is okay, dwelling on them is not productive. Nothing good comes from being submerged in guilt or shame. When struggling with these feelings, children may need help from their parents to recognize that mistakes are part of being human.

No one is perfect; nothing is perfect; and recovery is available, natural, and expected.

Similarly, parents may need to repair within themselves after a rupture with their children. Parents all make mistakes, and because their children are so precious to them, it can be hard to forgive themselves for mishandling them. After losing their temper with children, they may harbor feelings of guilt and shame. Parents may struggle to accept the reality that parenting is hard and that they will make mistakes.

Here is the perfect job for a family therapist: to help parents to find ways to forgive themselves, treat themselves compassionately, and get back on the path they have chosen. If not, parents can get stuck in their own emotional issues rather than being available for positive connections with their children.

RECONNECTION AND REPAIR

It is always parents' job to facilitate reconnection. This process is particularly critical if the disconnection is due to severe misbehavior or a slip back into parental harshness. When a rupture has occurred, parents can immediately convert the energy of interactions from negative back to positive. They can resume regular positive interaction and attention to children. They can move forward without recrimination, shaming, giving others the cold shoulder, or shutting down.

While parents may have the capacity to let go and move on, it is not appropriate to demand that children do the same. Let children have their feelings. Where children continue to simmer, stonewall, or recriminate about a past rupture, parents should respond neutrally—acknowledge the child's ongoing reaction without passion, energy, or defensiveness. Advise parents to avoid correcting children's angry feelings or arguing with them. Accepting that children may need more time to resolve their feelings is part of repairing and getting back on track. Research has found that chronic parental disconnection, if not repaired and shifted to a positive connection, will have detrimental effects on children's sense of self and relational trust, whereas parental reconnection and repair have positive effects on children's emotional and social development (Tronick, 2007, 2017).

When both parties are ready, it is important to reconnect. Reconnection can involve any combination of verbal, emotional, or physical interaction, including resuming fun, hugging, talking together, and reassuring children of their value and their parents' steady love. However, children must be ready and receptive toward attempts to repair. Finesse is needed; children must feel open to the type of reconnection parents are offering.

Within the context of a richly positive environment, repair can happen without a great need to discuss the rupture. In fact, dwelling on a past error can impede the repair process. Repair is complete when a steady stream of recognition and attention is unaffected by the rupture, causing the rupture to shrink in relative importance. As the energy of positive connection overcomes the echoes of the rupture, children have a real-time experience of security with parents who are forgiving, have confidence in them, and see them as lovable. This shift implies that mistakes are normal and that the moment of disconnection has passed.

If parents feel it is useful to discuss the rupture or if children bring it up, they can be encouraged to focus as much as possible on the success, not the error. They may say, "I noticed you stopped hitting," or "I see you yelled instead of hitting when you were angry." This style of mental processing allows children to move their emotional pain from implicit to explicit memory in a way that builds their positive regard for themselves. They become consciously aware of what happened and how they helped to resolve it. Having such a conversation with an emphasis on reviewing the entire course of errors and laying blame is not useful and can be counterproductive.

What parents communicate to their children with this approach is, "You are not the sum of your errors." You can coach parents to say this to themselves as well. Many adults are prone to guilt and self-recrimination, especially in the wake of a rupture with a child. A focus on failure is as counterproductive for helping adults build confidence and good parenting habits as it is for building self-confidence in their children.

Encourage parents to apologize to children where it seems called for. Apologies from parents to children are not a sign of weakness, but a sign of thoughtfulness and strength. They do not, however, replace adults taking responsibility for their behavior and taking action to prevent similar issues in the future. In a healthy process of sincere repair, children learn that their feelings matter even when parents are stressed or unhappy.

Our discussion of repair and reconnection brings us back to the start of our book: the integration of attachment security, emotional regulation, and learning through the parent–child relationship. As parents work to spend more time in emotional stability—and to repair and reconnect when they slip—they offer a secure base and a robust model for relationships for children. Moments when those slips occur can teach about recovery and forgiveness. No one is perfect: not parents, not children, and not therapists. There is always room for learning and growth.

CONCLUSION: RELATIONSHIP-BASED DISCIPLINE

Discipline problems are not simply caused by children and their behaviors. Rather, they are created in the context of the family and the environment in which the children are raised. Our therapeutic approach to discipline is designed to avoid escalation of negativity for both parents and children, and to maximize opportunities for attunement, learning, cooperation, and fun. In working with parents we prioritize the creation of a nurturing and responsive home, which is the fertile ground that children need to develop self-regulation and social acumen.

Parents are biologically driven to want to know what to do when their children misbehave. Our brains are problem-solving machines that are reliable in their search for trouble and their urge to dive into it and solve it. However, when it comes to parenting, discipline is not limited to times of trouble, but rather is baked into the moment-by-moment interactions of parents and children over time. When on track, parents ideally build a reliably secure and affirming context for children's lives. As children learn what is valued and honored in them, their choices begin to drift toward embodying their assets more and more consistently. This is the basis of discipline: reinforcing their inherent cooperation and positivity. Times of trouble do not have the potential for teaching that parents often hope for; however, they are important times for communicating to children where the limits are, and that no great fun or reward results from misbehavior or dysregulation.

Ideally, neurobiologically based and attachment-sound discipline serves to meet the 7 essential attachment needs. Using our relationship-based discipline approach with a balance of recognition and reset, clear rules, and parent regulation meets this goal. It provides children safe feedback about themselves that is soothing, attuned, consistent, encouraging, and fun, while simultaneously providing structure and boundaries.

In order to approach this goal, it is important for parents to commit to and practice their own emotional and behavioral regulation. To this end, our work with parents is necessarily deeper than mere parent consultation. It includes fostering self-awareness, creating a space for reflection, and placing a premium on parents taking mindful responsibility for their own feelings and actions. It is a delicate path to take, involving humility and self-evaluation. When parents take this journey, it can literally change the trajectory of their families' lives. The final destination is well worth the effort.

Conclusion: Integration of Relationship-Based Treatment

Relationship-based parenting is integrative parenting. It is not working independently with neurobiology, attachment, emotion, or discipline that creates powerful change for children, but rather an integrated approach that simultaneously takes its power from all of these (Figure C.1). Each of these areas, while independent, is also interdependent; they foster and build on one another. Even when we are pulled to discuss emotions, for example, we are always doing so while keeping in mind the attachment needs of the child, the innate neurobiology of all humans, and the family's typical discipline practices. Essentially, these cannot be broken apart; they are intrinsically linked at all times.

The innate neurobiology each individual carries through life is the raw material we work with in psychotherapy. It sets the stage for a child's sensitivities, capacities, and special needs, dictates our species-specific developmental need for care, and primes children and their parents for the attachment relationship. Our knowledge of neurobiology prepares us to understand what we are seeing in families such as their hardwired need for connection, struggles with emotion regulation, and tendency to repeat relational patterns as learned in the family.

In practical terms, understanding human neurobiology and the

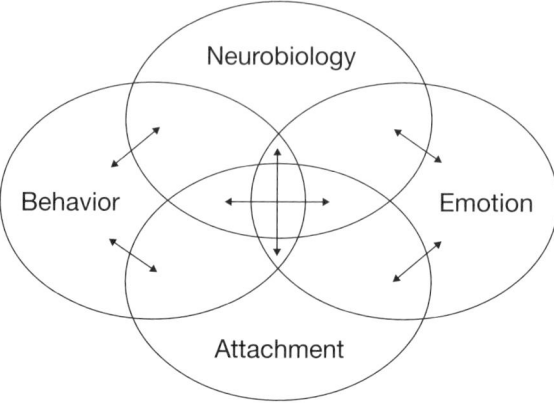

Figure C.1   Integrative Parenting

neurobiological development of children sets us up as therapists to be attuned and effective. Our grasp of the human nervous system helps us use interventions that are compatible with our patients' wiring. It helps us avoid interventions that may sound nice in theory but are destined to fail because they do not respect the neurobiological requirements of development, safety, and readiness to learn. When we help parents understand how their brains and nervous systems work, they can apply this science to build their own effective strategies for managing themselves and their children. Children can benefit from this knowledge also.

Although the human attachment system is neurobiologically based, it is also socially influenced—an intimate interweave of nature and nurture. An individual's attachment strategy guides their expectations of others, as well as their relationship tendencies and capabilities. It has a hearty influence on one's emotional experiences and regulation and influences a sense of self, confidence, and expectations of one's self. In family therapy, we are working with the nascent attachment system of the child, the established attachment systems of the parents, and, of course, our own attachment system. It is necessary, as a therapist, to have a good understanding of attachment science in order to navigate the thicket of unconscious relational impulses in any therapy room. This understanding prepares us to sensitively approach clients in a way that is comfortable to them, and to assist them in interacting with one another in ways that are considerate of one another's makeup. Finally, an important part of case conceptualization and treatment planning is noting where any of the 7 essential attachment needs are not being met, and bolstering them.

Neurobiology and attachment experiences lay the groundwork for each individual's emotional makeup. The resulting patterns of emotional awareness and expression are different for every person, and problems in this system are some of the most common concerns presented in family therapy. Our understanding of the interface of children's innate neurobiology and temperament, as well as their parent–child attachment patterns and the current family milieu, provide insight into the emotional world of the family. Children's developmental need for coregulation and inability to autonomously regulate is the basis of our work and important for parents to understand. With discernment, we can notice parental responses to children's emotions, such as the tendency to escalate, dismiss, or attune, which points to where work is needed. Parents' work often begins with learning to mindfully notice and accept their child's emotional state, even if the expressive behavior is not appropriate.

Refining parents' skills in responding compassionately to a child's feelings while still holding limits firmly is the gold standard. In order to reach this standard, parents must first be aware of and accept their own feelings. As therapists, a similar mindful stance—being present with and accepting of emotion rather than jumping to solutions—is the heart of emotional wisdom and fosters the same strength in parents. This backdrop enables us to create a therapeutic relationship with both parents and children that is soothing, attuned, and safe enough to allow for the vulnerability that can lead to growth. Increased emotional capacity benefits both children and parents in terms of their own comfort, as well as the health of their social and familial relationships.

When the referral question for a child is not emotion regulation, it is always behavior. Behavioral issues can emanate from how a child's innate neurobiology is responded to in the family system and are often closely tied to the parent–child attachment status and emotional state. Relationship-based discipline simultaneously soothes the emotional state of the child, fosters secure attachment, and is neurobiologically sound. It taps into children's natural drive to learn and emotionally connect with others. This type of parenting is responsive rather than punitive, and is initiated by reframing discipline away from behavioral control and toward finding success. Teachable moments—moments when the child is showing any glimmer of success—become the currency of discipline within this relationship-based approach.

A prerequisite of this intervention is parental competence at maintaining their own regulation and attunement to their child, which positions parents to effectively influence behavior without doing harm. At its core, relationship-based discipline holds that the child is inherently good and that growth can occur without disciplinary practices that wound the parent–child relationship. Relationship-based discipline offers a kind, hopeful approach to parents that is not merely philosophical but also provides concrete strategies for addressing behavior problems.

Our hope is that this integrated perspective, and the concrete steps you can take to work within it, will provide you with the knowledge and tools required to do the vital work of supporting and guiding families. It is our belief that as we therapists grow our mastery in these areas, we increase our effectiveness, and ultimately our confidence, joy, and energy in doing our important work. We wish you a sense of professional competence and fruitfulness, and we hope we have contributed to that.

References

Ainsworth, M. D., Blehar, M. C., Waters, E., & Wall, S. (1978). *Patterns of attachment: A psychological study of the strange situation*. Erlbaum.

Ainsworth, M. D., & Eichberg, C. (2006). Effects on infant-mother attachment of mother's unresolved loss of an attachment figure, or other traumatic experience. In C. M. Parkes, J. Stevenson-Hinde, & P. Marris (Eds.), *Attachment across the life cycle*. Routledge.

American Psychological Association. (2011). Children and trauma: Update for mental health professionals. Presidential Task Force on Posttraumatic Stress Disorder and Trauma in Children and Adolescents. https://www.apa.org/pi/families/resources/children-trauma-update.aspx

Andersen, S. L. (2003). Trajectories of brain development: Point of vulnerability or window of opportunity? *Neuroscience and Biobehavioral Reviews, 27*(1–2), 3–18.

Ang, E., & Gomez-Pinilla, F. (2007). Potential therapeutic effects of exercise to the brain. *Current Medicinal Chemistry, 14*(24), 2564–2571.

Austin, E., Saklofske, D., & Egan, V. (2005). Personality, well-being and health correlates of trait emotional intelligence. *Personality and Individual Differences, 38*(3), 547–558.

Badenoch, B. (2008). *Being a brain-wise therapist: A practical guide to interpersonal neurobiology*. Norton.

Bakermans-Kranenburg, M. J., Van Ijzendoorn, M. H., & Juffer, F. (2005). Disorganized infant attachment and preventative interventions: A review and meta-analysis. *Infant Mental Health Journal, 26*(3), 191–216.

Bakermans-Kranenburg, M. J., & van IJzendoorn, M. H. (2009). The first 10,000 adult attachment interviews: Distributions of adult attachment representations in clinical and non-clinical groups. *Attachment and Human Development, 11*(3), 223–263.

Balocchini, E., Chiamenti, G., & Lamborghini, A. (2013). Adolescents: Which risks for their life and health? *Journal of Preventative Medicine and Hygiene, 54*(4), 191–194.

Bastian, V., Burns, N. R., & Nettelbeck, T. (2005). Emotional intelligence predicts life skills, but not as well as personality and cognitive abilities. *Personality and Individual Differences, 39*(6), 1135–1145.

Baylin, J., & Hughes, D. A. (2016). *The neurobiology of attachment-focused therapy: Enhancing connection and trust in the treatment of children and adolescents.* Norton.

Berking, M., & Schwarz, J. (2014). Affect regulation training. In J. J. Gross (Ed.), *Handbook of emotional regulation.* Guilford.

Blair, C. (2008). Maternal and child contributions to cortisol response to emotional arousal in young children from low-income, rural communities. *Developmental Psychology, 44*(4), 1095.

Booth, P., & Jernberg, A. (2009). *Theraplay: Helping parents and children build better relationships through attachment-based play* (3rd ed.). Jossey-Bass.

Bowlby, J. (1951). Maternal care and mental health. *Bulletin of the World Health Organization, 3*, 355–533.

Bowlby, J. (1952). *Maternal care and mental health: A report prepared on behalf of the World Health Organization for the welfare of homeless children.* Palais des Nations, Geneva.

Bowlby, J. (1969). *Attachment and loss: Vol. 1. Attachment.* Basic Books.

Brazelton, T. B., & Greenspan, S. (2001). *The irreducible needs of children: What every child must have to grow, learn, and flourish.* Da Capo.

Brazelton, T. B., & Sparrow, J. (2006). *Touchpoints: Your child's emotional and behavioral development.* Da Capo Lifelong.

Broad, W. J. (2012). *The science of yoga: The risks and rewards.* Simon and Schuster.

Brody, G., Beach, S. R. H., Philibert, R., Chen, Y., Lei, M., Murry, V., & Brown, A. (2010). Parenting moderates a genetic vulnerability factor in longitudinal increases in youths' substance use. *Journal of Consulting Clinical Psychology, 77*(1), 1–11.

Brody, G., Yu, T., Chen, Y., Kogan, S. M., Evans, G., Windle, M., Gerrard, M., Gibbons, F., Simons, R., & Philibert, R. (2013). Supportive family environments, genes that confer sensitivity, and allostatic load among rural African American emerging adults: A prospective analysis. *Journal of Family Psychology, 27*(1), 22–29.

Brown, D. P., & Elliott, D. S. (2016). *Attachment disturbances in adults: Treatment for comprehensive repair.* Norton.

Brunk, M, A., Henggeler, S. W., & Whelan, J. P. (1987). Comparison of multisystemic therapy and parent training in brief treatment of child abuse and neglect. *Journal of Consulting and Clinical Psychology, 55*(2), 171–178.

Burke, C. A. (2010). Mindfulness-based approaches with children and adolescents: A preliminary review of current research in an emergent field. *Journal of Child and Family Studies, 19*, 133–144.

Burns, D. (2008). *Feeling good: The new mood therapy.* Harper.

Byrne, J. (2019). Cellular and molecular neurobiology. In *Neuroscience online: An electronic textbook for the neurosciences.* University of Texas Health Science Center. https://nba.uth.tmc.edu/neuroscience/m/index.htm.

Caldji, C., Diorio, J., & Meaney, M. J. (2000). Variations in maternal care in infancy regulate the development of stress reactivity. *Biological Psychiatry, 48*(12), 1164–1174.

Carrion, V., & Wong, S. (2012). Can traumatic stress alter the brain? Understanding the implications of early trauma on brain development and learning. *Journal of Adolescent Health, 51*(2), S23–S28.

Cassani, D. (2015). When mindfulness meets the classroom. *Atlantic Monthly,* August 31.

Cassidy, J., Jones, J. K., & Shaver, P. R. (2013). Contributions of attachment theory and research: A framework for future research, translation, and policy. *Developmental Psychopathology, 25*(4, Pt 2), 1415–1434.

Centers for Disease Control and Prevention. (2021). Violence prevention: Adverse childhood experiences. (April 2, 2021). Retrieved from https://www.cdc.gov/violenceprevention/aces/index.html

Chen, E., Miller, G., Yu, T., & Brody, G. (2018). Unsupportive parenting moderates the effects of family psychosocial intervention on metabolic syndrome in African American youth. *International Journal of Obesity, 42*(4), 634–640.

Chess, S., & Thomas, A. (1984). *Origins and evolution of behavior disorders.* Harvard University Press.

Coatsworth, J. D., Duncan, L. G., Greenberg, M. T., & Nix, R. L. (2009). Changing parent's mindfulness, child management skills and relationship quality with their youth: Results from a randomized pilot intervention trial. *Journal of Child and Family Studies, 19*(2), 203–217.

Cohen, A., Mannarino, A., & Deblinger, E. (2017). *Treating trauma and traumatic grief in children and adolescents* (2nd ed.). Guilford.

Cousins, N. (1991). *The celebration of life: A dialogue on hope, spirit and the immortality of the soul.* Bantam.

Cozolino, L. (2014). *The neuroscience of human relationships: Attachment and the developing social brain* (2nd ed.). Norton.

Cramer, S., Sur, M., Dobkin, B., O'Brien, C., Sanger, T., Trojanowski, J., Rumsey, J., Hicks, R., Cameron, J., Chen, D., Chen, W., Cohen, L., deCharms, C., Duffy, C., Eden, G., Fetz, E., Filart R., Freund, M., Grant, S., . . . Vinogradov, S. (2011). Harnessing neuroplasticity for clinical applications. *Brain, 134*(6), 1591–1609.

Crist, J. (2004). *What to do when you're scared and worried: A guide for kids.* Free Spirit.

Darwin, C. (2011). *The expression of the emotions in man and animals.* Appleton. (Original work published 1899)

David Lynch Foundation. (n.d.). *The Quiet Time Program: Restoring a positive culture of academics and well-being in high-need school communities.* San Francisco Unified School District.

Davidson, R. J., & McEwen, B. S. (2012). Social influences on neuroplasticity: Stress and interventions to promote well-being. *Nature Neuroscience, 15*(5), 689–695.

Deblinger, E., & Heflin, A. H. (1996). *Treating sexually abused children and their nonof-fending parents: A cognitive-behavioral approach.* Sage.

Derapelian, D. (2015). *Core attachment therapy: Secure attachment for the adopted child.* CreateSpace.

Dobbs, D. (2009). The science of success. *The Atlantic,* December.

Dubuc, B. (2013). The brain from top to bottom. *The Brain,* March.

Duncan, L. G., Coatsworth, J. D., & Greenberg, M. T. (2009). Pilot study to gauge acceptability of a mindfulness-based, family-focused preventive intervention. *Journal of Primary Prevention, 30*(5), 605–618.

Easterbrooks, M. A., Biesecker, G., & Lyons-Ruth, K. (2010). Infancy predictors of emotional availability in middle childhood: The roles of attachment security and maternal depressive symptomatology. *Attachment and Human Development, 2*(2), 170–187.

Epel, E. S., Blackburn, E. H., Lin, J., Dhabhar, F. S., Adler, N. E., Morrow, J. D., & Cawthon, R. M. (2004). Accelerated telomere shortening in response to life stress. *Proceedings of the National Academy of Science of the United States of America, 101*(49), 17312–17315.

Farb, N. A., Anderson, A. K., Irving, J. A., & Segal, Z. V. (2014). Mindfulness interventions and emotion regulation. In J. J. Gross (Ed.), *Handbook of emotion regulation.* Guilford.

Field, T. (2014). *Touch.* MIT Press.

Field, T., Diego, M., Hernandez-Reif, M., Deeds, O., & Figueiredo, B. (2009). Pregnancy massage reduces prematurity, low birth weight, and postpartum depression. *Infant Behavior and Development, 43*(4), 454–460.

Fischer, M. (2017). Mindfulness practice with children who have experienced trauma. *Master of Social Work Clinical Research Papers.* https://sophia.stkate.edu/msw_papers/736

Fisher, B., Petzinger, G., Nixon, K., Hogg, E., Bremmer, S., Meshul, C., & Jakowec, M. (2004). Exercise-induced behavioral recovery and neuroplasticity in the 1-methyl-4-phenyl-1,2, 3,6-tetrahydropyridine-lesioned mouse basal ganglia. *Journal of Neuroscience Research, 77*(3), 378–390.

Flaherty, A. W., & Rost, N. S. (2011). *The Massachusetts General Hospital handbook of neurology.* Lippincott Williams.

Fonagy, P., Gergely, G., Jurist, E., & Target, M. (2010). *Affect regulation, mentalization, and the development of the self.* Other Press.

Fosha, D., Siegel, D., & Solomon, M. (2009). *The healing power of emotion: Affective neuroscience, development and clinical practice.* Norton.

Fredrickson, B. (2013). *Love 2.0: Creating happiness and health in moments of connection.* Penguin.

Germer, C., Siegel, R., & Fulton, P. (2016). *Mindfulness and psychotherapy* (2nd ed.). Guilford.

Ginott, H., Ginott, A., & Goddard, W. (2003). *Between parent and child: The bestselling classic that revolutionized parent–child communication.* Harmony.

Glasser, H., & Easley, J. (2016). *Transforming the difficult child: The nurtured heart approach.* Nurtured Heart.

Glasser, H., & Lowenstein, M. (2017). *The transforming the intense child workbook.* Nurtured Heart.

Goodman, T. (2016). Working with children: A beginner's mind. In C. K. Germer, R. D. Siegel, & P. R. Fulton (Eds.), *Mindfulness and psychotherapy.* Guilford.

Greenberg, M., Cicchetti, D., & Cummings, E. M. (Eds.). (1990). *Attachment in the preschool years: Theory, research and intervention.* Chicago: Chicago University Press.

Greenberg, M. T., & Harris, A. R. (2012). Nurturing mindfulness in children and youth: Current state of research. *Child Development Perspectives, 6*(2), 161–166.

Gross, J. J. (Ed.). (2014). *Handbook of emotion regulation.* Guilford.

Gyurak, A., & Etkin, A. (2014). A neurobiological model of implicit and explicit regulation. In J. J. Gross (Ed.), *Handbook of emotion regulation.* Guilford.

Hackman, D. A., Betancourt, L. M., Brodsky, N. L., Kobrin, L., Hurt, H., & Farah, M. (2013). Selective impact of early parental responsivity on adolescent stress reactivity. *PLOS ONE, 8*(4).

Harrison, L. J., Manocha, R., & Rubia, K. (2004). Sahaja yoga meditation as a family treatment program for children with attention deficit-hyperactivity disorder. *Clinical Child Psychology and Psychiatry, 9*(4), 479–497. doi:10.1177/1359104504046155

Heinicke, C. M., Fineman, N. R., Ruth, G., Recchia, S. L., Guthrie, D., & Rodning, C. (1999). Relationship-based intervention with at-risk mothers: Outcome in the first year of life. *Infant Mental Health Journal, 20*(4), 349–374.

Hektner, J. M., Brennan, A. L., & Brotherson, S. E. (2013). A review of the Nurtured Heart approach to parenting: Evaluation of its theoretical and empirical foundations. *Family Process, 52*(3), 425–439.

Heller, S. (1997). *The vital touch: How intimate contact with your baby leads to happier, healthier development.* Owls Books.

Helliwell, J., Layard, R., & Sachs, J. (Eds.). (2017). *World happiness report 2017.* Sustainable Development Solutions Network.

Hietanen, J., Glerean, E., Hari, R., & Nummenmaa, L. (2016). Bodily maps of emotions across child development. *Developmental Science, 19*(6), 1–8.

Hoffman, K. T., Marvin, R. S., Cooper, G., & Powell, B. (2006). Changing toddlers' and preschoolers' attachment classifications: The circle of security intervention. *Attachment and Human Development, 74*(6), 1017–1026.

Huebner, D. (2005). *What to do when you worry too much: A kid's guide to overcoming anxiety.* Magination Press.

Hughes, D. (2007). *Attachment-focused family therapy.* Norton.

Hughes, D. (2011). *Attachment-focused family therapy workbook.* Norton.

Huizink, A., Robles de Medina, P. G., Mulder, E. J. H., Visser, G., & Buitelaar, J. K. H. (2003). Stress during pregnancy is associated with developmental outcome in infancy. *Journal of Child Psychology and Psychiatry, 44*(6), 810–818.

Hutt, R. L., Buss, K. A., & Kiel, E. J. (2012). Caregiver protective behavior, toddler fear and sadness, and toddler cortisol reactivity in novel contexts. *Infancy, 18* 708–728.

Iacoboni, M. (2009). Imitation, empathy, and mirror neurons. *Annual Review of Psychology, 60,* 653–670.

Juffer, F., Struis, E., Werner, C., & Bakermans-Kranenburg, M. (2017). Effective preventive interventions to support parents of young children: Illustrations from the video-feedback intervention to promote positive parenting and sensitive discipline (VIPP-SD). *Journal of Prevention and Intervention in the Community, 45*(3), 202–214.

Kabat-Zinn, J. (1982). An outpatient program in behavioral medicine for chronic pain patients based on the practices of mindfulness meditation: Theoretical considerations and preliminary results. *General Hospital Psychiatry, 4*(1), 33–47.

Kabat-Zinn, J. (2005). *Wherever you go, there you are: Mindfulness meditation in everyday life.* Hyperion.

Kabat-Zinn, J. (2018). *Meditation is not what you think: Mindfulness and why it is so important.* Hachette Books.

Kabat-Zinn, J., Massion, A., Kristeller, J., Peterson, L., Fletcher, K., Pbert, L., Linderking, W., & Santoelli, F. (1992). Effectiveness of a meditation-based stress reduction program in the treatment of anxiety disorders. *American Journal of Psychiatry, 149*(7), 936–943.

Kagan, J. (1998). *Galen's prophecy: Temperament In human nature.* Westview Press.

Karen, R. (1998). *Becoming attached: First relationships and how they shape our capacity to love.* Oxford University Press.

Karr, A. (1853). *Lettres écrites de mon jardin.* Publisher Michel Lévy Frères, Paris.

Keys, D. (1982). "The politics of consciousness." In *Earth at omega: Passage to planetization.* Branden Press. Boston, Massachusetts.

Kiecolt-Glaser, J. K., Gouin, J. P., Weng, N., Malarkey, W. B., Beversdorf, M. Q., & Glaser, R. (2010). Childhood adversity heightens the impact of later-life caregiving stress on telomere length and inflammation. *Psychosomatic Medicine, 73*(1), 16–22.

Kiff, C., Lengua, L., & Zalewski, M. (2011). Nature and nurturing: Parenting in the context of child temperament. *Clinical Child and Family Psychology Review, 14,* 251–301.

Kinver, M. (2013). Early life care shapes African elephant's future. *BBC News, Science and Environment,* February 13.

Konrath, S., Chopik, W., Hsing, C., & O'Brien, E. (2014). Changes in adult attachment style in American college students: A meta-analysis. *Personality and Social Psychology Review, 18*(4), 326–348.

Langer, E. (2016). *Power of mindful learning.* Da Capo Lifelong.

Laska, K. M., Gurman, A. S., & Wampold, B. E. (2014). Expanding the lens of evidence-based practice in psychotherapy: A common factors perspective. *Psychotherapy: Theory, Research, Practice, Training, 51*(4), 467–481.

Lazar, S. (2016). Mindfulness research. In C. K. Germer, R. D. Siegel, & P. R. Fulton (Eds.), *Mindfulness and psychotherapy.* Guilford.

Lazar, S. W., Kerr, C. E., Wasserman, R. H., Gray, J. R., Greve, D. N., Treadway, M. T., McGarvey, M., Quinn, B. T., Dusek, J. A., Benson, H., Rauch, S. L., Moore, C. I., Fischl, B. (2005). Meditation experience is associated with increased cortical thickness. *Neuroreport, 16*(17), 1893–1897.

Lee, J., Nader, K., & Schiller, D. (2017). An update on memory reconsolidation updating. *Trends in Cognitive Sciences, 21*(7), 531–545.

Lee, P., Bussiere, L., Webber, E., Poole, J., & Moss, C. (2013). Enduring consequences of early experiences: 40 year effects on survival and success among African elephants. *Journal of Biology Letters, 9*(2), 20130011.

Lester, B., & Sparrow, J. (Eds.). (2010). *Nurturing children and families: Building on the legacy of T. Berry Brazelton.* Wiley-Blackwell.

Levendosky, A., Huth-Bocks, A., Semel, M., & Shapiro, D. (2002). Trauma symptoms in preschool-age children exposed to domestic violence. *Journal of Interpersonal Violence, 17*, 150–164.

Levine, P. (2015). *Trauma and memory: Brain and body in a search for the living past.* North Atlantic Books.

Lippard, E., & Nemeroff, C. (2020). The devastating clinical consequences of child abuse and neglect: Increased disease vulnerability and poor treatment response in mood disorders. *American Journal of Psychiatry, 177*(1), 20–36.

Lite, L. (1996). *A boy and a bear.* Specialty Press/A.D.D. Warehouse.

Luerssen, A., & Ayduk, O. (2014). The role of emotion and emotion regulation in the ability to delay gratification. In J. J. Gross (Ed.), *Handbook of emotion regulation.* Guilford.

Lundahl, B., Nimer, J., & Parsons, B. (2006). Preventing child abuse: A meta-analysis of parent training programs. *Research on Social Work Practice, 16*(3), 251–262.

Main, M. (1990). Cross-cultural studies of attachment organization: Recent studies, changing methodologies, and the concept of conditional strategies. *Human Development, 33*, 48–61.

Main, M. (2006). Metacognitive knowledge, metacognitive monitoring, and singular (coherent) vs. multiple (incoherent) models of attachment. In C. M. Parkes, J. Stevenson-Hinde, & P. Marris (Eds.), *Attachment across the life cycle.* Routledge.

Main, M., & Hesse, E. (1990). Parents' unresolved traumatic experiences are related to infant disorganized attachment status: Is frightened and/or frightening parental behavior the linking mechanism? In M. Greenberg, D. Cicchetti, & E. M. Cummings (Eds.), *Attachment in the preschool years: Theory, research and intervention*. University of Chicago Press.

Main, M., & Solomon, J. (1990). Procedures for identifying infants as disorganized/disoriented during the Ainsworth Strange Situation. In M. T. Greenberg, D. Cicchetti, & E. M. Cummings (Eds.), *Attachment in the preschool years: Theory, research, and intervention*. University of Chicago Press.

Mate, G (2010). *In the realm of hungry ghosts: Close encounters with addiction*. North Atlantic Books.

May, R. (1963). "Freedom and responsibility re-examined." In E. Lloyd-Jones and E. Westervelt (Eds.) *Behavioral science and guidance: Proposals and perspectives*. Teachers College, Columbia University Press.

McClowry, S. G., Rodriguez, E. T., & Koslowitz, R. (2008). Temperament-based intervention: Re-examining goodness of fit. *European Journal of Developmental Science*, *2*(1–2), 120–135.

McEwen, B. (2005). Stressed or stressed out: What is the difference? *Journal of Psychiatry and Neuroscience, 30*(5), 315–318.

McGilchrist, I. (2012). *The master and his emissary: The divided brain and the making of the western world*. Yale University Press.

McGreevy, S. (2011). Eight weeks to a better brain. *Harvard Gazette*, January 21.

Medina, J. (2010). The genetics of temperament: An update. *Psychiatric Times, 27*(3).

Medina, J. (2014). *Brain rules for baby: How to raise a smart, happy child from zero to five*. Pear Press.

Menon, V., & Uddin, L. Q. (2010). Saliency, switching, attention and control: A network model of insula function. *Brain Structure and Function, 214*(5), 655–667.

Merrick, M., Ford, D., & Guinn, A. (2018). Prevalence of adverse childhood experiences from the 2011–2014 Behavioral Risk Factor Surveillance System in 23 states. *Journal of American Medical Association Pediatrics, 172*(11), 1038–1044.

Mesulam, M. (1999). Neuroplasticity failure in Alzheimer's disease: Bridging the gap between plaques and tangles. *Neuron, 24*(3), 521–529.

Middlebrooks, J. S., & Audage, N. C. (2008). *The effects of childhood stress on health across the lifespan for Disease Control and Prevention*, National Center for Injury Prevention and Control.

Mischel, W. (1958). Preference for delayed reinforcement: An experimental study of a cultural observation. *Journal of Abnormal and Social Psychology, 56*(1), 57–61.

Mischel, W. (2014). *The marshmallow test: Mastering self-control*. Little, Brown Spark.

Mischel, W., & Shoda, Y. (1988). The nature of adolescent competencies predicted by preschool delay of gratification. *Journal of Personality and Social Psychology, 54*(4), 687–696.

Moullin, S., Waldfogel, J., & Washbrook, E. (2018). Parent–child attachment as a mechanism of intergenerational (dis)advantage. *Families, Relationships and Societies, 7*(2), 265–284.

Nachmias, M., Gunnar, M., Mangelsdorf, S., Hornik Parritz, R., & Buss, K. (1996). Behavioral inhibition and stress reactivity: The moderating role of attachment security. *Child Development, 67*(2), 508–522.

Nakazawa, D. J. (2015). *Childhood disrupted.* Atria.

Naumburg, C. (2019). *How to stop losing your sh*t with your kids: A practical guide to becoming a calmer, happier parent.* Workman.

Nhat Hanh, T. N. (2019). *At home in the world: Stories and essential teaching from a monk's life.* Parallax.

Nummenmaa, L., Glerean, E., Hari, R., & Hietanen, J. (2014). Bodily maps of emotions. *Proceedings of the National Academy of Sciences of the USA, 111*(2), 646–651.

Nuño, V. L., Wertheim, B. C., Murphy, B. S., Glasser, H., Wahl, R. A., & Roe, D. J. (2020). The online nurtured heart approach to parenting: A randomized study to improve ADHD behaviors in children ages 6–8. *Ethical Human Psychology and Psychiatry, 22*(1), 31–48.

Ogden, P., & Fisher, J. (2015). *Sensorimotor psychotherapy: Interventions for trauma and attachment.* Norton.

Ogden, P., Minton, K., & Pain, C. (2006). *Trauma and the body: A sensorimotor approach to psychotherapy.* Norton.

Paddock, C. (2016). Exercise in pregnancy "good for mom and baby." *Medical News Today,* July 10. http://www.medicalnewstoday.com/articles/311531.php

Palmer, B., Donaldson, C., & Stough, C. (2002). Emotional intelligence and life satisfaction. *Personality and Individual Differences, 33*(7), 1091–1100.

Panksepp, J., & Biven, L. (2012). *The archaeology of mind: Neuroevolutionary origins of human emotions.* Norton.

Parkes, C. M., Stevenson-Hinde, J., & Marris, P. (Eds.) (2006). *Attachment across the life cycle.* Routledge.

Pennebaker, J. W. (2004). *Writing to heal: A journal for recovering from trauma and trauma emotional upheaval.* New Harbinger.

Petzinger, G., Holschneider, D., Fisher, B., McEwen, S., Kintz, N., Halliday, M., Toy, W., Walsh, J. W., Beeler, J., & Jakowec, M. W. (2015). The effects of exercise on dopamine neurotransmission in Parkinson's disease: Targeting neuroplasticity to modulate basal ganglia circuitry. *Brain Plasticity, 1*(1), 29–39.

Porges, S. (2011). *The polyvagal theory: Neurophysiological foundations of emotions, attachment, communication, and self-regulation.* Norton.

Porges, S. (2017). *The pocket guide to the polyvagal theory: The transformative power of feeling safe.* Norton.

Porges, S., & Furman, S. (2012). The early development of the autonomic nervous system provides a neural platform for social behavior: A polyvagal perspective. *Infant Child Development*, *20*(1), 106–118.

Posner, M., Tang, Y., & Lynch, G. (2014). Mechanisms of white matter change induced by meditation training. *Frontiers in Psychology*, *5*, 1220.

Raser, J. (2003). *Raising children you can live with: A guide for frustrated parents*. Bayou.

Robertson, J., & Robertson, J. (Directors) (1952). *A two-year-old goes to hospital* [Film]. Robertson Films.

Roelofs, K. (2017). Freeze for action: Neurobiological mechanisms in animal and human freezing. *Philosophical Transactions of the Royal Society of London, Series B Biological Sciences*, *372*(1718).

Rothenberg Gritz, J. (2015). Mantras before math class. *Atlantic Monthly*, November 10.

Sapolsky, R. (2004). *Why zebras don't get ulcers*. Holt Paperbacks.

Saunders, R., Jacobvitz, D., Zaccagnino, M., Beverung, L. M., & Hazen, N. (2011). Pathways to earned-security: The role of alternative support figures. *Attachment and Human Development*, *13*(4), 403–420.

Schab, L., & Myer, A. (1996). *The coping skills workbook: Teaches kids nine essential skills to help deal with real life crisis*. Childswork/Childsplay.

Schetter, C., & Tanner, L. (2012). Anxiety, depression, and stress in pregnancy: Implications for mothers, children, research, and practice. *Current Opinion in Psychiatry*, *25*(2), 141–148.

Schore, A. (2001). The effects of early relational trauma on right brain development, affect regulation, and infant mental health. *Infant Mental Health Journal*, *22*(1), 201–267.

Schore, A. (2012). *The science of the art of psychotherapy*. Norton.

Schore, A. (2015). *Affect regulation and the origin of the self: The neurobiology of emotional development*. Psychology Press.

Schore, A. (2017). Modern attachment theory. In S. N. Gold (Ed.), *APA handbook of trauma psychology: Foundations in knowledge*, 389–406. American Psychological Association.

Shaver, P. R., & Mikulincer, M. (2014). Adult attachment and emotion regulation. In J. J. Gross (Ed.), *Handbook of emotion regulation*. Guilford.

Shoda, Y., Mischel, W., & Peake, P. K. (1990). Predicting adolescent cognitive and self-regulatory competencies from preschool delay of gratification: Identifying diagnostic conditions. *Developmental Psychology*, *26*, 978–986.

Shonkoff, J., Garner, A., & the Committee on Psychosocial Aspects of Child and Family Health. (2012). The lifelong effects of early childhood adversity and toxic stress. *Pediatrics*, *129*(1), 232–246.

Siegel, D. (2015). *Brainstorm: The power and purpose of the teenage brain*. Tarcher/Penguin.

Siegel, D. J. (1999). *The developing mind: How relationships and the brain interact to shape who we are* (1st ed.). Guilford.

Siegel, D. J. (2020). *The developing mind: How relationships and the brain interact to shape who we are* (3rd ed.). Guilford.

Siegel, D. (2017). *Mind: A journey to the heart of being human.* Norton.

Siegel, D. J., & Bryson, T. (2012). *The whole-brain child: 12 revolutionary strategies to nurture your child's developing mind.* Bantam.

Siegel, D. J., & Hartzell, M. (2013). *Parenting from the inside out: How a deeper self-understanding can help you raise children who thrive* (10th anniv. ed.). Tarcher Perigee.

Singleton, O., Hölzel, B. K., Vangel, M., Brach, N., Carmody, J., & Lazar, S. W. (2014). Change in brainstem gray matter concentration following a mindfulness-based intervention is correlated with improvement in psychological well-being. *Frontiers in Human Neuroscience, 8*(33). doi:10.3389/fnhum.2014.00033

Snyder, J. S., Soumier, A., Brewer, M., Pickel, J., & Cameron, H. A. (2011). Adult hippocampal neurogenesis buffers stress responses and depressive behaviour. *Nature, 476*, 458–461.

Spear, L. P. (2013). Adolescent neurodevelopment. *Journal of Adolescent Health, 52*(2, Suppl. 2), S7–S13.

Spitz, R. (Director). (1952). *Emotional deprivation in infancy* [Film].

Sreenivasan, H. (2017). Faced with outsized stresses, these Baltimore students learn to take a deep breath." *PBS Newshour*, February 21. https://www.pbs.org/newshour/show/faced-outsized-stresses-baltimore-students-learn-take-deep-breath

Stegemoller, E. (2014). Exploring a neuroplasticity model of music therapy. *Journal of Music Therapy, 51*(3), 211–227.

Strauch, B. (2004). *The primal brain: What the new discoveries about the teenage brain tell us about our kids.* Bantam Doubleday.

Suomi, S. (2005). Mother-infant attachment, peer relationships, and the development of social networks in rhesus monkeys. *Human Development, 48*, 67–79.

Taffel, R., & Blau, M. (2002). *Parenting by heart.* Da Capo.

Taylor, K., Seminowicz, A., & Davis, K. (2008). Two systems of resting-state connectivity between the insula and cingulate cortex. *Human Brain Mapping, 30*(9), 2731–2745.

Teicher, M. H., Andersen, S. L., Polcari, A., Anderson, C. M., Navalta, C. P., & Kim, D. M. (2003). The neurobiological consequences of early stress and childhood maltreatment. *Neuroscience and Biobehavioral Reviews, 27*(1–2), 33–44.

Teicher, M. H., Samson, J. A., Anderson, C. M., & Ohashi, K. (2016). The effects of childhood maltreatment on brain structure, function, and connectivity. *Nature Reviews Neuroscience, 17*, 652–666.

Thoits, P. (2010). Stress and health: Major findings and policy implications. *Journal of Health and Social Behavior*, October 8.

Thompson, R. A. (2014). Socialization of emotion and emotion regulation in the family. In J. J. Gross (Ed.), *Handbook of emotion regulation*. Guilford.

Tiemeier, H., Lenroot, R., Greensein, D., Tran, L., Pierson, R., & Giedd, J. (2010). Cerebellum development during childhood and adolescence: A longitudinal morphometric MRI study. *Neuroimage*, *49*(1), 63–70.

Todeschin, A. S., Winkelmann-Duarte, E. C., Jacob, M. H., Aranda, C., Jacobs, S., Fernandes, M. C., Ribeiro, M. F., Sanvitto, G. L., & Lucion, A. B. (2009). Effects of neonatal handling on social memory, social interaction, and number of oxytocin and vasopressin neurons in rats. *Hormones and Behavior*, *56*, 93–100.

Toth, S., Rogosch, F., Manly, J., & Cicchetti, D. (2006). The efficacy of toddler-parent psychotherapy to reorganize attachment in the young offspring of mothers with major depressive disorder: A randomized preventive trial. *Journal of Consulting and Clinical Psychology*, *74*(6), 1006–1016.

Tough, P. (2012). *How children succeed: Grit, curiosity, and the hidden power of character*. Houghton Mifflin.

Tronick, E. (2007). *The neurobehavioral and social-emotional development of infants and children*. Norton.

Tronick, E. (2017). The caregiver–infant dyad as a buffer or transducer of resource enhancing or depleting factors that shape psychobiological development, *Australian and New Zealand Journal of Family Therapy*, *38*(4), 561–572.

US Department of Health and Human Services. (2014). *Child maltreatment*. www.acf .hhs.gov/sites/default/files/cb/cm2014.pdf

US Department of Health and Human Services. (2019). *Child abuse and neglect*. Child Welfare Information Gateway. http://www.childwelfare.gov/topics/can/

Vance, D., Roberson, A., McGuinness, T., & Fazeli, P. (2010). How neuroplasticity and cognitive reserve protect cognitive functioning. *Journal of Psychosocial Nursing and Mental Health Services*, *48*(4), 23–30.

Vandell, D., Belsky, J., Burchinal, M., Steinberg, L., & Vandergrift, N. (2010). Do effects of early child care extend to age 15 years? Results from the NICHD Study of Early Child Care and Youth Development. *Child Development*, *81*(3), 737–756.

van der Kolk, B. (2015). *The body keeps the score: Brain, mind, and body in the healing of trauma*. Penguin.

van der Put, C., Assink, M., Gubbels, J., & Boekhout van Solinge, N. (2018). Identifying effective components of child maltreatment interventions: A meta-analysis. *Clinical Child and Family Psychology Review*, *21*(2), 171–202.

van de Weijer-Bergsma, E., Formsma, A., De Bruin, E., & Bögels, S. (2012). The effectiveness of mindfulness training on behavioral problems and attentional functioning in adolescents with ADHD. *Journal of Child and Family Studies*, *21*(5), 775–787.

Vlahovicova, K., Melendez-Torres, G., Leijten, P., Knerr, W., & Gardner, F. (2017). Parenting programs for the prevention of child physical abuse recurrence: A systematic review and meta-analysis. *Clinical Child and Family Psychology Review*, *20*(3), 351–365.

Wallin, D. (2007). *Attachment in psychotherapy*. Guilford.

Wampold, B. (2017). *Qualities and actions of effective therapists*. American Psychological Association.

Waters, E., Weinfield, N., & Hamilton, C. (2000). The stability of attachment security from infancy to adolescence and early adulthood: General discussion. *Child Development*, *71*(3), 703–706.

Weissman, M., Leckman, J., Merikangas, K., Gammon, G., & Prusoff, B. (1984). Depression and anxiety disorders in parents and children results (Yale Family Study). *Archives of General Psychiatry, 41*(9), 845–852.

Whaley, S. E., Pinto, A., & Sigman, M. (1999). Characterizing interactions between anxious mothers and their children. *Journal of Consulting and Clinical Psychology*, *67*(6), 826–836.

Whiteman, H. (2017). Massaging your partner can boost your well-being, reduce stress. *Medical News Today*, May 6.

Williams, M., Teasdale, J., Segal, Z., & Kabat-Zinn, J. (2007). *The mindful way through depression*. Guilford.

Wilson, A. (2013). Mindfulness meditation and the brain. *Huffington Post*, February 19. https://www.huffpost.com/entry/mindfulness-meditation-brain_n_2680087

Winnicott, D. (1953). Transitional objects and transitional phenomena—a study of the first not-me possession. *International Journal of Psycho-Analysis, 34*, 88–97.

Winnicott, D. W. (1992). *The child, the family, and the outside world*. Penguin. (Original work published 1964)

Wolfson, A., Lacks, P., & Futterman, A. (1992). Effects of parent training on infant sleeping patterns, parents' stress and perceived parental competence. *Journal of Consulting and Clinical Psychology, 60*, 41–48.

Index

About the Authors

Elizabeth Sylvester, PhD, is a clinical psychologist working with children and their families in Austin, Texas for over 30 years. She is an advanced trainer of the Nurtured Heart Approach, and integrates this approach with her expertise in relational attachment and interpersonal neurobiology. She specializes in treating highly behaviorally and emotionally intense children and adolescents, combining parent interventions and psychotherapy. Dr. Sylvester is a cofounder of the Heart & Work series of writings and presentations, and of Austin Child Therapy, an organization whose mission is to support the work of pediatric mental health professionals. She is married and is the mother of twin sons.

Kat Scherer, PhD, MFT, C-IAYT, is a psychologist, educator, and speaker. She practices in Austin, Texas and presents on topics such as interpersonal neurobiology, emotional development, and the application of mindfulness in mental health. Her presentations have been offered in academic settings, professional conferences, and community settings. Dr. Scherer is a cofounder of Austin IN Connection, a multidisciplinary organization focused on emotional health and attachment. She cohosts the Heart & Work Series with two collaborative mental health blogs: Therapy Matters and Heart & Work of Parenting. She is also a former Brazelton Touchpoints trainer and a faculty member at the Practice School of Yoga Therapy.